INFORMATION TECHNOLOGY STRATEGIES FROM THE UNITED STATES AND THE EUROPEAN UNION

Studies in Health Technology and Informatics

Editors

Volume 76

Earlier published in this series

Vol. 45. J. Dudeck, B. Blobel, W. Lordieck and T. Bürkle (Eds.), New Technologies in Hospital Information Systems
Vol. 46. U. Gerdin, M. Tallberg and P. Wainwright (Eds.), Nursing Informatics
Vol. 47. W. Ceusters, P. Spyns, G. De Moor and W. Martin (Eds.), Syntactic-Semantic Tagging of Medical Texts: The Multi-TALE Project
Vol. 48. J. Graafmans, V. Taipale and N. Charness (Eds.), Gerontechnology
Vol. 49. L. van den Broek and A.J. Sikkel (Eds.), Health Cards '97
Vol. 50. J.D. Westwood, H.M. Hoffman, D. Stredney and S.J. Weghorst (Eds.), Medicine Meets Virtual Reality
Vol. 51. J. Mantas (Ed.), Advances in Health Telematics Education
Vol. 52. B. Cesnik, A.T. McCray and J.-R. Scherrer (Eds.), MedInfo '98
Vol. 53. M.C. Sievert, D.E. Moxley, N.J. Ogg and T.B. Patrick, Thesaurus of Health Informatics
Vol. 54. O. Ferrer-Roca and M. Sosa-Iudicissa (Eds.), Handbook of Telemedicine
Vol. 55. H.M.J. Goldschmidt, M.J.T. Cox, R.J.E. Grouls, W.A.J.H. van de Laar and G.G. van Merode, Reference Information Model for Clinical Laboratories
Vol. 56. I. Iakovidis, S. Maglavera and A. Trakatellis (Eds.), User Acceptance of Health Telematics Applications
Vol. 57. J. Mantas (Ed.), Health and Medical Informatics Education in Europe
Vol. 58. G. Riva, B.K. Wiederhold and E. Molinari (Eds.), Virtual Environments in Clinical Psychology and Neuroscience
Vol. 59. I.A.F. Stokes (Ed.), Research into Spinal Deformities 2
Vol. 60. M. Di Rienzo, G. Mancia, G. Parati, A. Pedotti and A. Zanchetti (Eds.), Methodology and Clinical Applications of Blood Pressure and Heart Rate Analysis
Vol. 61. R.A. Mortensen (Ed.), ICNP® and Telematic Applications for Nurses in Europe
Vol. 62. J.D. Westwood, H.M. Hoffman, R.A. Robb and D. Stredney (Eds.), Medicine Meets Virtual Reality
Vol. 63. R. Rogers and J. Reardon, Recommendations for International Action
Vol. 64. M. Nerlich and R. Kretschmer (Eds.), The Impact of Telemedicine on Health Care Management
Vol. 65. In production
Vol. 66. In production
Vol. 67. J. Oates and H. Bjerregaard Jensen (Eds.), Building Regional Health Care Networks in Europe
Vol. 68. P. Kokol, B. Zupan, J. Stare, M. Premik and R. Engelbrecht (Eds.), Medical Informatics Europe '99
Vol. 69. In production
Vol. 70. J.D. Westwood, H.M. Hoffman, G.T. Mogel, R.A. Robb and D. Stredney (Eds.), Medicine Meets Virtual Reality 2000
Vol. 71. J.T. Ottesen and M. Danielsen (Eds.), Mathematical Modelling in Medicine
Vol. 72. I. Iakovidis, S. Maglavera and A. Trakatellis (Eds.), User Acceptance of Health Telematics Applications
Vol. 73. In production
Vol. 74. In production
Vol. 75. In production

ISSN: 0926-9630

Information Technology Strategies from the United States and the European Union

Transferring Research to Practice for Health Care Improvement

Edited by

E.A. Balas

European Union Center, Center for Health Care Quality, University of Missouri, Columbia, MO, USA

S.A. Boren

Center for Health Care Quality, University of Missouri, Columbia, MO, USA

and

G.D. Brown

Department of Health Management and Informatics, University of Missouri, Columbia, MO, USA

IOS Press

Ohmsha

Amsterdam • Berlin • Oxford • Tokyo • Washington, DC

ISBN 1 58603 054 X (IOS Press)
ISBN 4 274 90347 8 C3047 (Ohmsha)
Library of Congress Catalog Card Number: 00-100288

Publisher
IOS Press
Van Diemenstraat 94
1013 CN Amsterdam
The Netherlands
fax: +31 20 620 3419
e-mail: order@iospress.nl

Distributor in the UK and Ireland
IOS Press/Lavis Marketing
73 Lime Walk
Headington
Oxford OX3 7AD
England
fax: +44 1865 75 0079

Distributor in the USA and Canada
IOS Press, Inc.
5795-G Burke Centre Parkway
Burke, VA 22015
USA
fax: +1 703 323 3668
e-mail: iosbooks@iospress.com

Distributor in Germany
IOS Press
Spandauer Strasse 2
D-10178 Berlin
Germany
fax: +49 30 242 3113

Distributor in Japan
Ohmsha, Ltd.
3-1 Kanda Nishiki-cho
Chiyoda-ku, Tokyo 101
Japan
fax: +81 3 3233 2426

PRINTED IN THE NETHERLANDS

Introduction

While clinical and biomedical research production is rapidly growing, delivery to practitioners remains unacceptably slow. Numerous studies document significant delay, loss, and waste in the production and dissemination of evidence from research. To improve health care quality and to make the best scientific achievements part of usual practices, clinicians have to be informed. Better information systems and services are needed to support health care practices in absorbing and efficiently introducing the constantly growing amount of information. There is a need for a more systematic analysis of practical relevance and better overall efficiency in the process of transferring clinical evidence from research to practice.

The purpose of this book is to provide insight into the new and innovative uses of computers and other digital information technologies from European and American leaders in the fields of communication and health information sciences. Information technologies are impacting organizations, communities and societies and redefining systems for education, work, health services and almost every other aspect of life. Throughout the book the issues of how information technologies can facilitate health care quality improvement by transferring research evidence to practitioners is explored through emerging information technologies, better information for quality health care, and international collaboration. The book is divided into three sections, with several chapters in each section.

The first section describes the information infrastructure for transferring research. New scientific information is being discovered at a rapid rate. Putting research into practice should be the ultimate goal of emerging information technologies. The chapter by Donald A.B. Lindberg, M.D. of the National Library of Medicine addresses the transfer of research through high performance computing. Literature-based and fact-based services that help deliver modern scientific information at the time and place that it is most useful are discussed. Otto Rienhoff, M.D. of the Georg August University in Göttingen, Germany provides an overview of how the training and delivery of medical care needs to be reengineered. Medical training is not keeping up with modern realities. Doctors need to be trained to deal with more informed patients and information technologies. Physician practices need retooling to deal with the isolation many physicians feel in their everyday practices. A high degree of specialization, massive information flow, and better-informed patients create a desire among physicians to link to other physicians. Ilias Iakovidis, Ph.D. of the European Commission on Telecommunications in Brussels, Belgium highlights European initiatives in the emerging health information infrastructure and citizen-centered shared care. The health information infrastructure is an enabling mechanism for continuity of care. Reed M. Gardner, Ph.D. of the University of Utah in Salt Lake City, Utah focuses on methods of gathering and using clinical data for clinical research and patient care. The examples in this chapter are based on the HELP hospital computer system at LDS Hospital in Salt Lake City.

The second section includes three chapters that describe aspects of how knowledge can be structured for practical application. Alexa T. McCray, Ph.D. of the Lister Hill National Center for Biomedical Communications which is part of the National Library of Medicine in Bethesda, Maryland provides an introduction to the digital libraries initiative funded by the U.S. federal government, a discussion of the Unified Medical Language System, and issues in creating Web-accessible resources for health care consumers. Nancy

M. Lorenzi, Ph.D. of the University of Cincinnati and Robert T. Riley, Ph.D. of Riley Associates in Cincinnati, Ohio discuss knowledge and change in health care organizations by focusing on the reality that managing change is crucial to the success of an information system. Users must be involved in systems development from the beginning to feel ownership in the system and look upon it as "our" system, not "their" system or "my" system. A successful project depends 80% on the social and political interaction skills of the developer and only 20% on implementation of the hardware and software. The developer must have organizational savvy, and be aware of who in the organization has the ability to make things happen, i.e., be "positively political." Jean Roberts, B.Sc. M.B.C.S., M.H.S.M., C.Eng. of First Consulting Group in Macclesfield, United Kingdom addresses how to incorporate knowledge into commercially available systems. This chapter focuses on attitudes to the transfer of knowledge, funding mechanisms and how to protect an investment in knowledge.

The third section deals with practical solutions to obtain better information for improved health care quality. Janet Corrigan, Ph.D., M.B.A. of the Institute of Medicine at the National Academy of Sciences in Washington, D.C. discusses the current state of health care quality and describes some of the factors that are hindering efforts to move toward evidence-based practice. The efforts of the President's Advisory Commission on Consumer Protection and Quality are also described. Kenneth D. Bopp, Ph.D. of University of Missouri in Columbia, Missouri highlights the multiple roles patients play in the health care process. Patients are both consumers and co-producers of services. Patients provide information that is critical to their diagnosis and treatment. They need to receive instructions on exactly what they are to do to carry out their treatment. Patients are banding together in self-help groups for their conditions, and giving input as to how they wish health professionals to deal with them. Mary Jane Richman, R.N., M.N., P.N.P. and Jeffrey S. Poltawsky, M.S., C.H.E. of Egleston Scottish Rite Children's Healthcare System in Atlanta, Georgia provide an example of how evidence-based disease management can be applied to a population of pediatric asthma patients to improve quality and access while decreasing total health care costs.

As mentioned earlier, international collaboration appears to be vital to move forward with efforts to prepare for modern practice and improve health care quality. However, various issues must be addressed between Europe and the United States in order to move forward with collaborations. The main challenges in transferring research to practice are user acceptance, cultural differences, national and regional strategies, legal and ethical issues, and standardization of technologies. We need to shift our attention to these enabling mechanisms for good implementation.

The degree of difference between the definitions of health professions in the various countries is quite dramatic. The same words are used, but they represent different legal concepts, professional roles, and self-understanding. For international collaboration to be successful, we need to recognize that we deal with hundreds of different professional types and not just with three or four. In countries that are in dire need of health professionals, differently educated health professionals may help fill that need.

A major stumbling block to future international collaboration is agreement on protection of medical data. The Council of Europe recommendations, issued in February 1997, do not carry the weight of law, but do highlight the need for serious dialogue between the European Union and United States. Information ethics research is needed to address medical ethics aspects of the use of databases.

This book comes out of the conference "Transferring Research to Practice in the Information Age" held at the University of Missouri, November 12 and 13, 1998. This two-day conference also coincided with the opening of the European Union Center at the University of Missouri.

E. Andrew Balas, M.D., Ph.D.
Suzanne Austin Boren, M.H.A.
Gordon D. Brown, Ph.D.

Acknowledgements

We thank the following groups and individuals for their support of the conference "Transferring Research to Practice in the Information Age" held in Columbia, Missouri, November 12–13, 1998 and this resulting publication:

- European Union Center at the University of Missouri
- Department of Health Management and Informatics at the University of Missouri
- Center for Health Care Quality at the University of Missouri
- Scientific Program Committee: E. Andrew Balas, M.D., Ph.D. (chair), Edward Brent, Ph.D., Gordon D. Brown, Ph.D., Cathleen Burns, Ph.D., Su-Shing Chen, Ph.D., Allen Hahn, D.V.M., Ph.D., Robert Logan, Ph.D., and Patricia Ramsay
- a grant from the U.S. National Library of Medicine (LM05545)

Contents

Introduction v
Acknowledgements viii

Information Infrastructure for Transferring Research

Transferring Research through High Performance Computing,
D.A.B. Lindberg 3
Retooling Practitioners in the Information Age,
O. Rienhoff 11
Towards a Health Telematics Infrastructure in the European Union,
I. Iakovidis 23
Interaction between Clinical Research and Patient Data,
R.M. Gardner 35

Structuring Knowledge for Practical Application

Digital Library Research and Application,
A.T. McCray 51
Knowledge and Change in Health Care Organizations,
N.M. Lorenzi and R.T. Riley 63
Incorporating Knowledge into Commercially Available Systems,
J. Roberts 71

Practical Solutions: Better Information for Improved Health Care Quality

Opportunities for Improving Quality in the Health Care Industry,
J.M. Corrigan 81
Information Services that Make Patients Co-Producers of Quality Health Care,
K.D. Bopp 93
Partnership for Excellence in Asthma Care: Evidence-Based Disease
Management, *M.J. Richman and J.S. Poltawsky* 107

Author Index 123

Information Infrastructure for Transferring Research

Information Technology Strategies from
the United States and the European Union
E.A. Balas et al. (Eds)
IOS Press 2000

Transferring Research Through High Performance Computing

Donald A.B. Lindberg, M.D.
Director, National Library of Medicine
Bethesda, Maryland, USA

1. Introduction

We tend to think, first there is research, then application. In fact, the two phases inform each other. Before there is either phase, matters of policy should be considered. In one sense, medical informatics may be viewed simply as a facilitator of research, a contributor to what other people do. But it really has a life in and of itself. If you look just at the facilitator role of medical informatics, one thinks, for example, of drill and practice training, simulation modeling, and transferring discoveries to practice. But because of the scholarly aspects of the field, medical informatics merits research [1]. It is acknowledge that the medical informatics field is roughly where molecular biology was 25 years ago. We do not yet know all the principles and we do not know the data generating sources the way we now understand genetics. Basic research is needed in computer graphics, imaging, knowledge representation and linking, and what used to be called "man-machine interface." This last could more accurately be termed interfacing information with a human user.

The University of Missouri is in a very good position to provide the environment for this interface. A few examples involve e-mail, support of basic research and clinical research, medical education, simulation and modeling, and transferring discoveries to practice.

Aside from word processing, electronic mail is by far the commonest computer application. It began with the ARPANET years ago. In fact, with an ARPANET account 20 years ago, one could communicate with other American universities and overseas with great ease. Although, it was sometimes easier to send a message to Japan than across campus.

ARPANET was basically an “elitist” research system, as was the subsequent National Research and Education Network of the High Performance Computing and Communications Initiative. The HPCC program was written up by then Senator Al Gore in 1989, and passed in 1991 and signed by President Bush. It was truly bipartisan in nature and, although I was tapped by President Bush to lead it, President Clinton and Vice President Gore strongly supported the program. Essentially, a communication system that would operate at a billion bits per second to link computers and the users was to be developed. A machine that would operate at a trillion floating point operations per second was wanted.

In 1989, this 5-year goal seemed unachievable, it was said, and if you actually had such a system, what would you do with it? In fact, it was accomplished in two-and-a-half years. The politicians did the right thing and began talking about democratizing it, and using Mr. Gore's phrase, “the electronic information highway.” Now we could begin to focus on applications.

We are seeing the success of the Internet in no small measure because of the HPCC: its $1.2 billion per year investments have made quite a difference. It is worth noting that TCP/IP, the Internet protocol, was developed not by a government agency or a corporation. This can be attributed to two individuals-Bob Kahn and Vincent Cerf. Everything that has happened since is a result of their scalable design. To understand where we go from here, you should be familiar with a couple of new terms: Next Generation Internet (NGI) and Global Information Infrastructure (GII). The NGI is funded at the level of a hundred million dollars a year, which would not be enough to design a whole new system were it not superimposed on the initial commitment. The UCAID, University Corporation for Advanced Information Development, essentially the university counterpart to the NGI which is basically composed of government agencies. The most public effort of UCAID is the new high speed communication network connections that link the various member universities to the National Science Foundation supported VBNS (very high speed backbone network service).

Global satellite systems are of increasing importance. Iridium, which has just been launched, will have 67 satellites. Another competitor is the GlobalStar System with 48 satellites, the Ellipso system with 16, and the Hughes system with 12. Why the great difference in satellites? The answer does not involve geometry or engineering; one need only know that the satellite “footprints” of some of the proposals cover only those countries and cities where the potential monetary return is greatest. You can get along with a smaller number of satellites if, in fact, the only place you're looking is where there is ready business. That is not a strategy that will give us a worldwide information society.

2. Literature-based Databases

Systems are needed that help deliver modern scientific information at the time and place that it is most useful. In medicine, that is with the patient and the physician, at the point of medical decision making. We at the National Library of Medicine (NLM) are responsible for MEDLINE, the premier bibliographic database of the health sciences literature, and GenBank, the enormous database of molecular sequences (http://www.nlm.nih.gov/.). There have been joking references to the growth of the medical literature by people who actually weigh the published Index Medicus. Index Medicus currently weighs several hundred pounds. When the weight of Index Medicus is graphed you will notice that the growth is linear and you might well ask, "Where is the information explosion?" The answer, quite simply, is in the specialized areas surrounding molecular biology, such as the mapped human genes and 3-D molecular data.

The MEDLINE database has exploded in usage. Heart Surgeon Michael E. DeBakey, a good friend of the NLM who has twice been on the Board of Regents, helped in the campaign to introduced free MEDLINE searching via the World Wide Web. The NLM was able to transition from fee-based to universal free searching because the Internet packet-based digital system had much greater efficiency than earlier analog telephony-based communication systems. This freed the NLM from the necessity of paying millions of dollars in telecommunications charges to the excellent but much less efficient value added service of the telephony-based common carriers. Free MEDLINE was launched in June 1997 at a press conference in Washington, D.C. Senators Arlen Specter (R, PA) and Tom Harkin (D, IA) and Vice President Gore all took part in making the announcement. The Vice President's remarks could not have been scripted better when he said, "I dare say that this development by itself may do more to reform and improve the quality of health care in the United States than anything else we've done in a long time." Since that announcement, the level of MEDLINE searching has skyrocketed from 7 million searches a year to more than 170 million. Equally as astonishing as the number of searches is who is doing the searching: 30 percent of the searches are being done by consumers (http://www.databases/freemedl.html.).

3. Fact-based Services

We turn now from the literature-based databases to fact based services. These fall primarily into two categories: molecular biology and toxicology/environmental health. The National Center for Biotechnology Information was created in 1988, the product of a formal long range planning process within the NLM and the intense interest in this subject in the Congress. The planning strategy was “bottom up.” In 1985, panels of people were assembled, and it was discovered that there was tremendous ferment in molecular biology. Labs were sequencing genes and a tremendous amount of data was being generated that would have benefit to all in the future, if it were carefully collected and shared. An organization to handle this was clearly needed, and the National Library of Medicine was the logical locus for the activity. Claude Pepper, the oldest man in the House of Representatives with some of the newest, and best ideas, wrote the legislation.

The National Center for Biotechnology Information. Under the leadership of Dr. David Lipman, has had a great influence on how research is done involving the human genome. The ENTREZ system, developed by the Center's scientists, is one such advance. It, and the broader GenBank systems, allow one to look at molecular biology sequence data in combination with MEDLINE. One can go from the published literature (MEDLINE) first to the nucleotide sequences that characterize DNA, then the protein products of those genes, then, after enough information is gathered, to the map of the genes on the chromosomes, and even, in many cases to the 3-dimensional structure of the protein product. It is the ability to link all these elements that is the real contribution of GenBank.

Using one article found in the literature, one could expand a search by asking for similar articles; similarly, in GenBank one can ask for DNA patterns that are similar and then link back to the articles that reported them. The most advanced version of the system links out to the gene expression data and also links to the full-text of articles of some MEDLINE journals. There are about 400 journals whose full-text articles are so linked at the present time, representing more than 70 publishers.

4. Linking Information

It is crucial that the information described remains linked, for when data gets "lost" the scientific process slows down. For example, Allen Cormack, the South African physicist, was given the Nobel Prize for inventing the CAT scan [2]. Geoffrey Houndsfield, who was an engineer at EMI ANGEL Records in England, made the machine itself. Cormack had published a design of the whole proposition 10 years before in the Journal of Applied Physics. I once introduced Cormack at a meeting and asked him about his discovery and how he did the mathematics basic to the system. "Oh well, I had to do much of the mathematics ab initio over about six years." He said, "Fourteen years would elapse before I learned that RADON (a French astronomer) had solved the [mathematical] problem in 1917." So there are the links: from the macrovision of looking at the heavens to (46 years later) the microvision of the CAT scan-the links are tenuous and almost did not get forged. The discovery was almost "lost."

5. Lister Hill National Center for Biomedical Communications

The staff of one of the research and development components, the Lister Hill National Center for Biomedical Communications, does some of the most important work of the NLM. One of their significant contributions is the development of the Unified Medical Language System [3]. Other work is being supported by NLM research grants, aimed at the development of the Electronic Patient Record, which has been much in the news these days. Patient records today should ideally be multimedia and contain images: one wants to be able to point and click and get X-rays, EKG's, images of tissue, even heart and breathing sounds. The Center has just taken on a new project to develop a comprehensive, Web-based, easy-to-use Clinical Trials Database. This database, which we are about to begin testing, will eventually contain information about clinical trials, both federally and non-federally funded, for experimental treatments for serious diseases and conditions. It should be a great boon to physicians and patients alike.

6. Telemedicine

The NLM is an enthusiastic sponsor of telemedicine, the exchange of medical information in support of remote decision making. The NLM is supporting a variety of "tele-" projects, many of them for populations that are underserved or have special needs such as rural and inner city areas, and the elderly. Here are a few examples: a nurse who makes "visits" to elderly patients via interactive TV and discusses their progress and problems, reviews their medication, and diet. She can "see" six or eight patients, in their homes, all before noon. Initially there was trepidation as to whether these experiments would be seen as a "Big Brother" intrusion into private lives. In fact, these older patients have embraced the technology with a remarkable enthusiasm. It makes them feel that somebody cares about them; they get up early and look forward to the sessions. Another specific example is in the setting of this rural physician's office, where the transmission of digital color images of a disabling skin condition led to a diagnosis by a university based dermatologist and a cure for the condition that the man had suffered for five years.

7. Visible Human Project

Perhaps the NLM research program that has resulted in the most publicity is the Visible Human Project [4]. The Visible Humans consist of two immense files totaling 55 gigabytes of data derived from carefully selected human cadavers-one male and one female. The datasets were prepared for NLM by scientists under contract at the University of Colorado using state-of-the-art radiographic (Computerized axial tomograph and magnetic resonance images) and photographic capture of cryosections. The NLM has awarded more than 1000 no-cost licenses to use the datasets to scientists in more than 30 countries. These creative researchers, physicians, and computer scientists are working with the Visible Humans in a number of exciting areas: teaching anatomy, modeling plastic and reconstructive surgery for individual patients, experimental "virtual colonoscopy", treatment planning that takes into account radiation absorption by the body, rehearsing prostate and other surgery, needle insertion simulation, and constructing ergonomic furniture, to name a few of the many applications now under development. A second Visible Human project has begun with several other NIH institutes, including the National Institute of Dental and Craniofacial Research, to create a high quality image set of the head and neck region. The visible human has spawned all kinds of good work. This project is proof that if you make a first class dataset, put it in the public domain, distribute it on Internet, you can fire the enthusiasm of hundreds of collaborators world wide.

8. National Heart Attack Alert Program

A new project that may have a direct payoff in lives saved is a collaboration of the National Heart, Lung, and Blood Institute with the NLM. The supposition is that if fibrinolytic agents are administered within an hour of a heart attack, many more patients would survive. Although the efficacy of these agents has been known for years, only a fraction of those suffering a heart attack receive this treatment. After a decade of trying to improve on this record, very little has changed. In 1997, fourteen awards were made under the rubric of the National Heart Attack Alert Program to see if researchers could apply medical informatics techniques to improve the situation. Here are some examples of the types of projects that have been funded: ambulances and helicopters sending EKG signals to the ER so that they are ready there with the optimum treatment when the patient arrives; toll-free telephone numbers for decision support for the patients; patient controlled medical records and self-referral schemes for chest pain; and wearable, intelligent monitoring devices.

9. Smartcards

The last topic I would like to touch on derives from my participation on behalf of the U.S. government in the G7 health related programs. One particular project, being carried out in France, Germany, and Italy, of interest to me is the smartcard project. This is an area in which Europe is way ahead of the U.S. Those countries have created a standard and have ordered tens of millions of these smartcards to be used in health care both by health care practitioners and by patients. The U.S. is participating in a small way in the smartcard program. The biggest past project in this country was one sponsored by the Department of Veterans Affairs-with 5000 participants. A new project is the Health Passport Project of the U.S. Western Governors Association. For some 22,000 women and their children these cards will contain pre-school immunization data and data for various health services such as Medicaid, Medicare, food supplementation, and immunizations. The amount of data that can be stored on the smartcard chips is yet to be determined; tens of thousands of the bits are sufficient for some basic medical purposes, although we may ultimately have millions available to us. We believe the US is ahead of Europe in the quality of our telecommunication system. Hence, we should be able to link our smartcards to remote information resources (e.g., URL codes to distant servers).

Computer intelligence has become “wearable.” In this case the computer intelligence is in a ring. The ring has the entire JAVA language, plus all of the encryption technology necessary to send, receive, decode and encrypt messages. You can build this capability into rings, you can put them on pencils, you can even put them on tee-shirts.

References

[1] Lindberg, D.A.B. High Performance Libraries. In: The British Library, Dainton Lectures on Scientific and Technical Information, London 1993.

[2] Cormack, A M. Early cat scanning and recent developments, part 1. In: Lindberg DAB, Kaihara S, eds. Proceedings of MEDINFO 80 Tokyo, Third World Conference on Medical Informatics, Amsterdam: North Holland Publishing Company, 1980: ix-xiii.

[3] Lindberg, D.A.B, Humphreys, B.L, McCray, A.T. The Unified Medical Language System. Meth Inform Med 1993; 32:281-291.

[4] Ackerman, M.J. The Visible Human Project: A resource for Education. Acad Med 74(6):667-670, 1999.

Information Technology Strategies from
the United States and the European Union
E.A. Balas et al. (Eds)
IOS Press 2000

Retooling Practitioners in the Information Age

Otto Rienhoff, M.D.
Professor & Chairman, Division of Medical Informatics
Georg August University
Göttingen, Germany

Abstract. For "retooling" one needs two components: new hardware and new skills. "Hardware" in the Medical Informatics environment includes not only hardware in a narrow definition, but operating and application software, network services, security services etc. Since the sixties, Medical Informatics has slowly moved from fighting computer hardware to fighting the complexity of application software and its installation. Thus the hardware part in the retooling process has changed but did not decrease in importance. Retooling medical professionals also means retraining of professionals - often a major investment. Regarding the necessary skills, we have to adapt existing medical curricula and continuous medical education (CME). So far, these have not successfully been adjusted to the retooling needs. The international community has to address these matters, specifically in the context of medical curriculum and CME.

1. The Tools

When you talk about *retooling* in the traditional sense, you always consider organizational and training aspects besides the technical tool itself. In the Middle Ages, it was well defined which craft (defined by tools) was allowed to do what. Correspondingly it was defined how the various professionals were trained. The medieval system regulated markets, and therefore made sure that an income was available for most professionals. Thus, already at that time training and organizational aspects were as important as the technical tools belonging to a craftsmanship. Today the question is: how do we have to organize the health informatics services as the computer has become a rather general tool in health care [1]. Typical questions are: Who is playing which role? How can specific application functions be guaranteed? How does one guarantee privacy? These issues are of increasing importance as we are advancing further into the information age and as computers and information services are available everywhere in the medical world. Maybe we need more specific legislation because the degree of change which we have to organize in medicine and health care is so high that codes of good practice are no longer sufficient to cope with its complexity. Information technology (IT) is changing the medical world and raises many questions [2, 3]. Some reasons why it may be necessary to retool the practitioners are summarized below.

2. Professional Isolation

Physicians in Germany, and in most parts of Europe, are often working in a professionally isolated situation, and they are aware of it. Three years ago, this fact was the reason for the elaboration of a national consultation paper on how to promote medical professional quality in Germany. It recommended a national curriculum containing a variety of personal and technical communication skills for all 300,000 German physicians [4].

The majority of doctors do not feel at ease in their professional isolation and would vountarily leave it. This isolation has nothing to do with their physical location, for example practices in the country-side versus medical faculty. Doctors are highly specialized, they experience a massive information flow, and they meet with increasingly well-informed patients. In this situation doctors would hail an exchange with other health professionals.

Information technology (IT) can network doctors, and other health professionals, and get them out of professional isolation - probably one of the biggest advantages in the retooling process. This is possible, so we ought to set out onto this way. The United States and many other countries are moving into this direction.

Examples exist how low-end-video communication systems based on a simple PC, which can be compared to an extension of the traditional telephone services, are well accepted in the medical field. They have led to a number of positive results, even under harsh economic conditions as could be proven in Norway, in Greece, but also in Germany with its extremely high density of physicians, and in the United States. Hence networking and low-end-telemedicine communication is definitely something which doctors can use. It helps medicine and health care in an economic way, and not only in sparsely populated countries like Canada or Australia with very few professionals, but also in regions with a high density of population like the centers of Europe.

3. Quality Management

Since the sixties, computer based quality assurance measures in medicine have been moved ahead (especially in the United States). From the work of Brook (Rand Corporation) and various projects in the seventies and eighties, we learned that quality management in medicine works, but needs continuous attention. However, we also know that it is costly and that it needs specific attitudes and skills of the health professionals. Europe has copied the US development, and as usual we are about ten years behind. We are currently in a phase of searching for new approaches to the question of quality management. One advantage of information technology is that we have the possibility to network doctors.

In Germany, "quality circles" (different from task-oriented US quality teams) are fashionable. Doctors are regularly brought together under a specific theme which they develop further into new fields of mutual interest. Along this line, but within a networked situation, one could define new ways of cooperation in quality management that were not available in the seventies: A feed-back circle could be built up between those physicians' groups working in the country in a more isolated situation and maybe professional groups of health care organizations, of physician chambers, or national provincial health advisory bodies. Thus, the latter could get some feed-back from the basic groups who work in the field, something that was not possible two decades ago.

Even if discussed and debated, evidence-based medicine is something we have to learn more about in the next decade. Some encouraging steps have already been taken into this direction in several Western countries.

4. Electronic Patient Records as a Starting Point

For many fields we know how to build up electronic patient records, but not for all. Although so far they have not been implemented in most countries, electronic patient records are something which will definitely come. However, right now the development still lacks globally successful products [5]. Electronic patient records are one of the reasons why we have to retool our health professionals.

5. Patient-Physician Relationship

In the patient-physician relationship the role of the patient is changing. Most dramatic changes have been effected through the availability of medical information for the lay-community and for the patient. One example: During the first year of free access to Medline, user rates increased by 30 percent, mainly because of non-professional requests. In a German government study on the development of these information services it was analyzed how the private and the public sector should act in this area. In Europe, most actors believe that information for the public is an inalienable and basic right, and this is true not only in the political arena, but also in health care. Therefore the information business is not left just to private companies. Some free and basic information services open to everyone also in the health care field and guaranteed by the public health administration in each specific country are envisaged.

6. Self-Help Groups

Many industrialized countries have witnessed a very strong development of self-help groups among patients using networked information systems. Though self-help groups can rely on a strong tradition in Germany, they never held the limelight except in very big issues, for example in the diabetes debate. Hundreds of minor issues never managed to attract public attention. However, this has changed dramatically over the last five years because those organizations have picked up new IT means. They have linked, not only on a national but also on an international level. Suddenly the self-help groups stand up and argue on conferences, they argue in the political scene, and they want to change the way health professionals are dealing with them and talk to them. Even the new German government mentioned this fact in its declaration of health policy last autumn.

One can also quote a dramatic example from Japan, where severely handicapped patients talk to each other by means of video communication. They feel free to communicate despite the fact that they are severely handicapped, maybe connected to a respirator or confined to their beds. Yet they can communicate with human beings who share their fate. It seems that patient-to-patient communication using video technique may experience a dramatic boom in the next years.

7. Telemonitoring

Besides the mentioned possibilities of networking, telemonitoring is also slowly coming up: Telemonitoring means that patients with a specific problem carry a device which is linked to e.g. a GSM system. The very moment a problem occurs, the system triggers off an alarm. Such systems will influence the doctor's professional work - the way he deals with emergency problems. Telemonitoring is quickly evolving. Interestingly, many systems are developed in Israel. A number of systems is developed with funds from the military arena.

8. Physicians' Responsibilities to be Redefined

Summing up all of these changes and new developments, maybe we have to redefine the way physicians deal with patients. If we retool the health professionals, if we retool the physician, is it the same physician that we had in mind some decades ago? Is it still the same physician who was, for example, described in the Flexner Reports in 1910? Is that the type of physician we are looking for or is it a different person?

The term "managed care" is not used so much in Europe; - we use "shared care." This is due to the fact that Europe's political and social background differs from that of the United States of America. Since managed care sounds a bit too commercial to us we rather talk about shared care, although there is the same idea behind both terms. Inter-professional collaboration is developing very much and very strongly in most countries. The problem for all of us is that this inter-professional collaboration is different from country to country.

The G7 studies about health data cards found out that the degree of difference between the definitions of health professions in various countries is quite dramatic. Only for very traditional professions like physicians and midwives, if you talk to someone in the UK, in Italy or in Germany, there is basically the same idea behind the legal definition of the specific responsibilities. However, if you move to any other profession, we use the same words, but they represent different legal concepts, different professional roles, self-image, and training. Therefore, if we move ahead with networking health professionals we have to bear in mind that on an international level, we are dealing with hundreds of different types of professionals, and not with three or four.

So if physicians, for example, are networked and perform telemedicine, they have to understand which capacity, which background, and which legal power their telemedical counterpart has. If this appears to be very simple - it is not! It is only easy for physicians in such countries that provide the same physicians' training. But, for example, it does not apply to many developing countries, because these have used the name of physicians to house different types of health professionals (barefoot doctors).

9. Handicapped or Elderly Patients in Augmented Care Reality Environments

Dave Warner is one of the famous people in the United States who has tried to help severely handicapped patients with computers and information technology. This idea is gaining ground on the European continent as we also try to develop systems that allow handicapped or elderly patients to live in augmented environments. One of the terms used in Europe to describe this development is the concept of the "intelligent home." First fairs deal with these questions, then a whole industry is build up.

This produces a new environment for the primary care professional. The doctors, the midwives, and the nurses are finding themselves in a different environment involving quality management, networked patients, and networked professionals. If we take all these factors into consideration, we know how much retooling is needed.

10. Complexity of Medicine

The growing complexity of medicine is not primarily due to the enormous rise of medical literature. Actually, I am very skeptical about that aspect. Unfortunately, we encounter so much worthless literature that the problem is rather one of selection than of assimilation. The dramatic increase in complexity is rather brought about by molecular medicine, which is trying first to understand and second to develop individualized treatments that are linked to our genetic definition.

If individualized treatment spreads in the future - and not only in pharmacological therapy, but also in radiation therapy and other therapies - then the way how we train physicians; operate medical services; do clinical work; carry out population studies in epidemiology; in short: all our activities in the health care sector will have to be re-engineered in relation to these results during in the next 10 to 30 years. It will be a fascinating task for our children. Although this is still ahead of us, it is starting to develop.

This means that we definitely have to retool the professionals who will enter the field in the next generation.

It also means that medicine is facing a generation of new scientific studies reanalyzing existing knowledge in relation to molecular information and adding huge quantities of new information. There will be no chance any more to just remember complex treatments as we are used to do it today. Computer support will be a must.

11. New Partners: Trusted Third Parties and Certification Bodies

We must guarantee for security of our communication systems, which means we have to find out how we can communicate using encryption techniques and how to digitally sign information. Information may also mean images or anything we wish to communicate to somebody else, including voice information. In our societies, we must be able to assign a legally accepted status to information accumulated in networks and computers. So far we have not been able to achieve this. Legal security is not only necessary in electronic commerce; it is also needed in medicine, maybe even more there. The technical concepts for trusted third party schemes (a term which you can write in various modes) have already been developed. These concepts may differ from each other, but at least they have been developed and do exist.

We absolutely need politicians who understand this issue. Politicians who understand that they have to develop policies and missions for our national governments to make telemedicine and telematics a legally accepted entity of the health care world. This is not something which doctors themselves can bring up. We need the political support as well as the support from legal community. And again, the constructs are there, but, at least in my country, for example, the Ministry of Health's staff does not include one person who is sufficiently knowledgeable about these issues. And why not? Because the ministry conceives the problem as relating to the electronic commerce business, therefore the Ministry of Interior would be responsible for it. I think this is a major problem that we all have to face right now.

The same problems arise with certification bodies. The Food and Drug Administration has very carefully tried to move into the direction of decision support systems evaluation and then carefully pulled out again. We do not have methodological approaches to certify some of the information systems that we have been discussing. But our patients will expect that there is some trustworthiness in equipment and information systems. So we have to move ahead in this field.

12. Continuous Medical Education (CME)

We need means to train doctors or other health professionals at home. They cannot be expected to be travelling all the time to sit in courses. There is a need for virtual practical cases to train them "on the job." We need to use IT to give them relevant information to train and work on, and to document their performance. And again, this has to be developed in line with privacy rules. It is the same idea as in other fields of quality management. We have to obtain performance data of the doctors, but at the same time use it to build up feed-back circles to orient continuous medical education towards the real needs of the doctors or the health professionals in the field. Some projects are currently dedicated to this purpose. They represent a very difficult, but urgent request.

13. New Professions and Shift of Professional Roles

A very, very difficult question is: Do we need new professions? For many of our traditional medical societies, this is a dangerous discussion. Much more than in America, doctors in Europe, specifically in the Northern parts, play a very dominant role in health care. They undergo a difficult process because information technology is questioning their professional hierarchies. Information technology is also questioning their roles in relation to other health professions and patients. Under this pressure many doctors react with a conservative approach. Many of them look backwards to the fifties or maybe even sixties when the world was better to physicians. However, we have to keep in mind a few examples of new approaches. For instance, the idea of the barefoot physician in China worked well. In many developing countries we find differently educated types of health professionals (e.g. primary health workers) with a status somewhere between a well-trained nurse and a doctor.

Let me also quote a famous example from the US military which specifically European doctors dislike very much. For several decades, the military had not been able to attract enough radiologists. Therefore it was not able to staff medical units worldwide with doctors who were specifically trained in this field. So the US military developed teleradiology to move all CT scans to the Veterans Administration which read them and sent the results back to the units worldwide. Though it was probably never designed this way, it became the first global experiment to redefine doctors and their role through information technologies, and it worked. In some European countries, professional organizations of doctors are redefining, not retooling, their professional role to prevent this sort of replacement. For example, the German pathologists' organization has set up a professional code that tries to prevent telepathology in Germany.

So we are dealing with a changing world and the questions of new professions are arising. In a recent meeting in Berlin somebody stated: "In this world of telemedicine, do we need a special profession, close to a doctor, but maybe not exactly a doctor, a profession specialized in dealing directly with patients by means of new communication devices?" I have no answer to that question, but it is one that we must discuss.

14. Skills for Tools - The Medical Curriculum

International experience has shown that the current training in medical schools is not addressing these matters. The curricula of Harvard University, McMasters University in Canada, and Maastricht University in The Netherlands are examples of change over the last ten years. However, most of these approaches have not been too successful. Internationally, many medical faculties are in a conservative mood since IT has created an insecurity within the establishment. Some even try to move backwards to restore the secure situation of the forties and fifties. This also happened in Germany. Over three years, intensive efforts were directed into a modernization of the medical curriculum. At the end of this attempt, a very conservative fraction of the national deans group managed to model the curriculum according to a very traditional design.

So we have to set out onto new ways of international collaboration in trying to define the medical curriculum for the next century - a major task that will take years to be done. As long as this job is not completed and consequently new curricula be implemented we still train the next generation of doctors for the traditional (non-IT) set of tools.

15. Enabling Technologies

A key aspect within the redefinition of curricula are the so-called "enabling technologies." These technologies (like 3D image manipulation) enable a young professional to perform his job at a most advanced level of know-how. Most American and

German physicians have been trained by working with cadavers. We still train medical students this way, although we know that most of them will do their practical work in a different environment. For example, over the last two to three years one could observe a dramatic change in the acceptance of robotic surgery by surgeons.

It seems that the most practical profession in the physician's world starts to accept computers as a support tool. The surgeons are still running the show, but computers support them. This means that their surgical work is no longer done only with their own hands. However, surgeons may have to develop new ways to work with image-guided systems, and even to relate their haptic feeling to images. This implies an entirely different type of training than in the traditional curriculum.

Results of general research on how doctors learn give hints on the difficulties to realize new curricular approaches [6, 7]. Those who have been involved in medical training know how difficult it is, for example, to teach ECG analysis to medical students, and how to link anatomical spatial relationships to what they see in the different tracings. So if they see a curve, what is really happening inside? When doctors or midwives learn to use their fingers to palpate a woman and to combine what they feel and see with their anatomical knowledge, this is a very complex training procedure. Some argue that if they once have been trained to do it the traditional way, then retraining of such professionals towards image-guided therapies is very difficult. Maybe because of our mode of learning, it is extremely difficult for us to retool ourselves if dramatic changes take place. More research is necessary in this context.

The medical curriculum is not sufficiently adapted to these new methods of dealing with patients and with information. So the spearhead of the health care service, the physicians, are still trained to work with tools of the last century. Maybe physicians will be that professional group which, for the longest time, tries to keep up the old situation, which would put them into direct contrast to the actual development. Such a disadvantageous scenario would doubtlessly have a major impact on the speed of development.

16. Market-Oriented Health Care Systems Versus Public Service-Oriented Systems

The health care systems of the world are very differently structured. The US system is market-oriented, and such a system primarily aims at efficiency. In the United States, most European systems are commonly called "socialistic", which is a simplified phrase for systems primarily aiming at coverage. These European public-service oriented health care systems tend to avoid costly IT-investments, even if politicians know that this is not the right way to look at new developments in health care [8]. However, it is felt that the implementation of computer tools with which one can retool doctors are very costly. As health administrations are primarily looking at technical developments from the public health point of view, the cost involved do not motivating to invest in IT. Instead, results of very difficult evaluations are requested before one moves ahead. So in many European countries health administration managers and key physicians are in agreement that the IT development is going too fast. As a result of this, the retooling of practitioners is lagging substantially behind.

17. Conclusion

The examples given show that the retooling of health professionals is urgently needed. However, not only the necessary financial investments into hardware are difficult to achieve, because of decreasing funds in health care. More substantially the retooling process is slowed down as the retraining of all professionals does not take place to any relevant degree. Even our schools of medicine focus on traditional ways of training the profession. For them and for the CME process new curricular models are needed - a substantial task comparable to the Flexner report early this century.

References

[1] Rienhoff, O. (1997). Can Medical Informatics Deliver? - How useful is the present communication infrastructure in Health Care? In L. van den Broek, Sikkel, A. J. (Eds.), *Health Cards '97 - Studies in Health Technology and Informatics* (Vol. 49, pp. 19-22). Amsterdam, Berlin, Oxford, Tokyo, Washington, DC: IOS Press.

[2] World Health Organization (1998). *A Health Telematics Policy in support of WHO's Health-for-All Strategy for Global Health Development.* Report of the WQHO Group Consultation on Health Telematics, December 11-16, Geneva, 1997.

[3] Sosa-Indicissa, M., Oliveri, N., Gamboa, C.A., Roberts, J. (Eds.), *Internet, Telematics and Health.* Amsterdam: IOS Press.

[4] Rienhoff, O., Brüggemann, M., Effer, E., Fischer, G. C., Knuth, P., Kolkmann, F.-W., Müller, W., Ollenschläger, G., Strobrawa, F.F. (1996). Curriculum Qualitätssicherung Teil 1: Ärztliches Qualitätsmanagement. Bundesärztekammer, Kassenärztliche Bundesvereinigung, Arbeitsgemeinschaft der Wissenschaftlichen Medizinischen Fachgesellschaften (Ed.), Köln: Bundesärztekammer.

[5] Rienhoff, O. (1994). Health Informatics Methodology and the Fragmented Health Care Market. In K. Brunnstein, Raubold, E. (Eds.), *Proceedings of the IFIP 13th World Computer Congress 94* (Vol. 2, pp. 494-501). Amsterdam: Elsevier Science B.V. North-Holland.

[6] Mantas, J. (Ed.)(1997). *Health Telematics Education.* Amsterdam: IOS Press.

[7] Cesnik, B., McCray, A.T., Scherrer, J.-R. (Eds.), *MEDINFO 98* (Vol. 1, pp. 197-201). Amsterdam: IOS Press.

[8] Rienhoff, O. (1997). The Health Informatics Wave and Decision Makers. In M. Sosa-Indicissa, Oliveri, N., Gamboa, C.A., Roberts, J. (Eds.), *Internet, Telematics and Health* (pp. 51-5). Amsterdam: IOS Press.

Information Technology Strategies from
the United States and the European Union
E.A. Balas et al. (Eds)
IOS Press 2000

Towards a Health Telematics Infrastructure in the European Union

Ilias Iakovidis, Ph.D.
Scientific Officer, European Commission, DGXIII
Brussels, Belgium

Abstract. Over the last decade information and communication technologies - telematics technologies - have demonstrated their potential to improve the quality, access and efficiency of health care. Health telematics applications are presently revolutionizing the developments not only in diagnosis, treatment, surveillance and rehabilitation of patients, but also on the side of the more collective aspects of health care and health prevention such as clinical trials, epidemiology and health education. Moreover, for the first time in the history of health care the emerging *Health Information Infrastructure (HII)*, i.e. telematics networks together with a set of technologies, health telematics applications and services, is making possible the rapid dissemination and sharing of health information and research results. This is leading to knowledge creation and to promotion of innovative approaches based on evidence collected in medical practice all over the world.

1. Introduction

Europe is actively participating in this revolution both through national strategic plans as well as European initiatives, such as the research and development programs of the European Union (EU). In 1985, the European Community launched a combined effort to formulate mid to long term strategy for Europe in the application of information and communication technologies to health care and biotechnology. An Exploratory Action was adopted by the Council in 1988 with a Community contribution of 20 million ECU (MECU). The Exploratory Action was followed in 1991 by the Advance Informatics in Medicine (AIM) Programme with a European Community contribution of 111 MECU. In 1993, the White Paper on Growth, Competitiveness and Employment stressed the need for a European information infrastructure as a tool for the creation of the "Information Society". The general preference in the United States, until recently, was for the term "Information Super-highways", implying a technology-based appreciation of current and future developments. By contrast, "Information Society" reflects European concerns about broader social and organizational changes and the quality of our lives, which will be delivered by the new information technologies.

We are presently at the end of the Fourth Framework Programme of Research Technological Development and Demonstrations (1994-1998) of the EU. The Telematics Applications Programme (TAP) is one of the larger programs (902 MECU, approximately 1 billion US dollars). One of the sectors of the Telematics Applications Programme is the Telematics Applications for Health (146 MECU). The main aim of the Telematics Applications for Health sector is to enable the entire health sector to benefit from the access to telematics applications and services. The emphasis in the last four years has been on user orientation and large validation of health telematics technologies leading the way to the establishment of a European HII. Some of the examples of products and services that are being developed in these projects include: multimedia patient records, interoperable health cards in a multilingual environment, multimedia quality assurance systems for cancer diagnosis and treatment, reference medical image databases, regional healthcare networks using standardized electronic data interchange (EDI) communication, 24 hour multilingual emergency telemedicine services for ships and remote areas, multimedia citizen advisory services for healthcare, multimedia training material and courses for health professionals. Information about these projects can be found at the web site of European Health Telematics Observatory Project of the Telematics Applications for the Health Sector of the European Commission (http://www.ehto.org).

In this chapter, we discuss the present prospects of the emerging European HII by describing its role as an enabling mechanism for continuity of care and focus on one of its most important components, the electronic health record. Finally, we will discuss the major challenges for the creation of a HII in the European Union.

2. Current Situation and Prospects

In the constant competition for resources in the health sector these new so-called telematics technologies and applications would not stand much chance if they were not intended to improve the quality of care, directly or indirectly, to help in cost-containment and better management of health sector, and to increase the competitiveness of the health telematics industry. Consequently, we should not forget that health information infrastructure can not be seen as a goal in itself but as an enabling mechanism for *continuity of care*. Here by the term continuity of care we mean continuous provision of health care through all the stages, namely prevention, diagnosis, treatment and rehabilitation, as well as continuity and collaboration across all the points of care such as hospitals, primary care centers, rehabilitation centers, labs, pharmacies, health authorities, homes, etc. with the individual (citizen) at the center. This citizen-centered care is a result of a growing trend for more effective management and the need for collaborative work of health professionals or in other words *shared care*. Under a shared care scheme we envision (i) health care professionals will collaborate and have access to relevant information in a timely and secure manner for decision support and research; (ii) managers and health authorities will have access to relevant information including information coming from both clinical and administrative data in order to make rational decisions; and (iii) citizens will have access to information enabling them to take a more active role in the process of disease prevention, health education, care and rehabilitation.

Shared care builds on a health information infrastructure linking hospitals, laboratories, pharmacies, primary care and social centers. Such an infrastructure has to accommodate not only the health professionals in the EU, i.e. 2.2 million nurses, 1.2 million physicians, 273,000 pharmacists and 200,000 dentists, but also 375 million EU citizens (1994 WHO data). Of course all the health-related information shared by all care providers, managers, industries and citizens must be comprehensive, reliable and confidential. For example the telemedicine services do not need to be isolated on a future HII but have access to relevant patient data stored elsewhere or to interact with other services of the HII (Figure 1).

It should be clear that although the HII focuses on one of the important application areas it does not drive the developments in the generic information and telecommunication infrastructure. The particularities of HII are best expressed in one of the four main application areas of HII, namely electronic health records [1]. The other three areas are population-based data, knowledge management and decision support, and telemedicine.

If the Healthcare Record is the collection of all the health-related information about an individual, then the Electronic Healthcare Record (EHR) is defined as a digitally stored (subset) of the Healthcare Record designed to support shared care, education and research. A distinction is made between the EHR and the EHR System that operates on the EHR in order to manage the information and provide information to qualified users in a user-friendly manner. The EHR system provides a virtual view of a patient record that is a

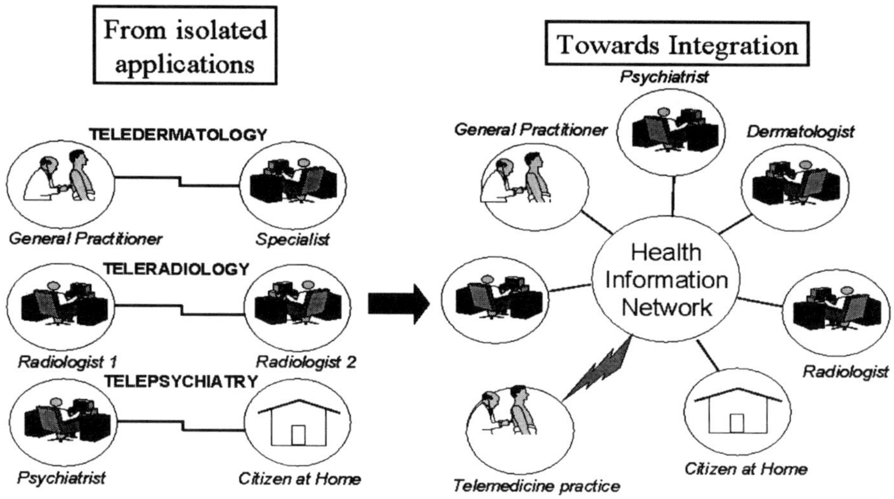

Figure 1: Example of Integration of Telemedicine Services

synthesis of data coming from a distributed system of interoperable databases. Such an EHR system can be implemented on different levels. It can support a group of physicians, or an enterprise, i.e. hospital and group of primary care clinics. Ideally it is implemented as a part of a regional health network connecting hospitals, primary care centers, rehabilitation centers, labs, pharmacies, health authorities, and homes and that way contributing to the shared care scenario described above. Good EHR systems help the users to retrieve the information in fast and user-friendly manner, to communicate easily with others, and make users work more effective. The EHR system must ensure confidentiality at all times by meeting all the security requirements.

The critical issues for the EHR, and consequently for the HII, are the standards regarding the record architecture, classification, terminology and coding. The common record architecture standard is a model of the generic features necessary in any EHR for it to be communicable and complete, retain integrity across systems, countries and time, and be a useful and effective ethical-legal record of care. In other words it is an agreed structure that can accommodate all types of data and support different views and at the same time preserve the meaning and the context. This standardized architecture should be a general model of the record so it can enable the development of many different systems with a particular instance of this architecture. Recently the Technical Committee TC251 of CEN (http://www.centc251.org/) has produced a draft pre-standard for the EHR architecture, which will be discussed at the level of each member state before adoption. The EC funded project dealing with these issues is EHCR-SupA (http://www.ehto.org or http://www.chime.ucl.ac.uk/HealthI/EHCR-SupA/). The standardized *terminology* is necessary to preserve the meaning, for proper coding of diseases and classification of medical procedures, for there to be any possibility of multilinguality or links and updates to other knowledge sources. The variety of medical concepts even within the same language make the classification and coding problems very difficult. There are efforts on the international level such as ICD, SNOMED, ICNP and NANDA for nursing and many more, but none of them is universally accepted and the mapping between them is difficult. Such mapping effort has started at the US National Library of Medicine. The work on terminology is long lasting and difficult and requires the concerted effort of many disciplines and countries. The relevant EU funded projects in this area are GALEN IN USE and TELENURSE (http://www.ehto.org).

The critical issues for EHR systems, and consequently for the HII, are the technological issues pertaining to storage, maintenance, communication and retrieval of multimedia information in different technological platforms and heterogeneous database systems that may be geographically distributed. The integration and interface of multivendor platforms and the development of health sector specific middleware and applications have recently received a lot of effort by research and development projects. The relevant EU funded projects are SYNAPSES, HANSA, I4C and SYNEX (http://www.ehto.org). Also large companies have many problems keeping the initial "legacy" systems running in the hospitals by interfacing them with new departmental systems and updating to new technologies. The standardization of the exchange format of course depends very much on the previous two categories, namely, the standards for architecture and terminology, since for access to the EHR and the "virtual" displaying of requested information one needs an object dictionary of terms and objects related to the structure and the terms in the record. There is a lot of progress expected using the Intranet approach for institutions and Internet based communications for the regions. There is also in parallel a large effort by the projects and standardization bodies in the area of Electronic Data Interchange (EDI) to standardize some particular messages, for example laboratory input/output, discharge letter communications between hospitals and physicians. Such EDI based communication has been demonstrated in the EU funded project COCO (http://www.ehto.org).

Other important attributes of EHR systems are the security and the standards for the security features such as digital signature, digital keys and other authentication systems. Most of the security applications and technologies are not health sector specific and the development is mainly pushed by the large financial or military institutions. The issues of security are closely related to the requirements of the confidentiality that is inherent in the definition of the EHR and will also be legally required by the national legislation. The relevant EU projects are TRUSTHEALTH and SIREN (http://www.ehto.org). There are many other important attributes such as accessibility and availability, reliability, usability, etc that one could list depending on the particular interest or use [2]. Next, let us examine the present situation in terms of implementation of EHR systems.

So far in hospitals, the most common information systems in use are the administrative and management hospital information systems. Not many hospitals in the world have information systems that integrate both clinical and administrative patient information and are sharable by different specialists and other health professionals. The first pilot projects are set up through European projects such as the hospitals involved in SYNEX, SYNAPSES and HANSA projects or through national efforts (e.g. in Greece where a large effort is under development to set up hospital information systems in 25 hospitals). As we have discussed above there is more to it than interfacing the existing system and setting up Intranets in hospitals. Due to the lack of standards on the conceptual work related to the architecture, terminology and communication there are still no true EHR systems as we have described them. However, there are many attempts that focus on particular features and functionalities. We will discuss the difficulties of setting up, and more importantly keeping up, such hospital based EHR systems in the next section.

The EHR systems or practice management systems for the general practitioner have, so far, the highest penetration. They are very popular in countries that have a strong tradition in primary care such as the United Kingdom, Ireland, Netherlands, Denmark and others. Figure 2 indicates the percentages of physicians using computers in their medical practice. The data is based on a study performed by the CAM Group in the 11 countries of Europe and supplementary data obtained by the author from health authorities of the different Member States [3].

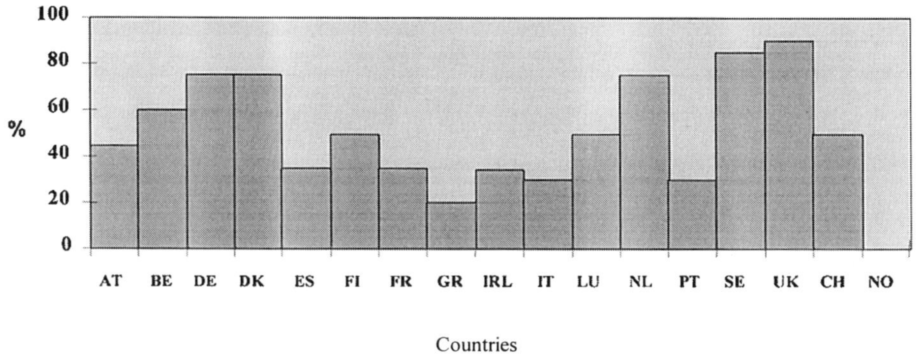

Figure 2: Percentage of Physicians Having Computers in their Practice

The percentages of physicians that are using clinical data on their computer or some form of EHR are normally much lower. A study in UK shows that the use of the software by general practitioners in UK is mainly for patient registration (98%) and repeat prescribing (94%). Only (29%) of general practitioners keep full clinical records electronically and only 14% have a "paperless office" [4]. The computerization and consequently use of electronic medical systems is growing rapidly in some European countries either because the GPs act as gatekeepers working alone or in small groups and it is easier to manage the systems (e.g. UK and Netherlands) or because of regulations and policies that require the physicians to submit reimbursement claims electronically (e.g. France). Moreover, the decision of some countries to distribute patient health cards requires the physicians to buy a card reader and a computer (e.g. Germany). Finally, the use of electronic medical records in primary care is much higher in Europe compared to anywhere in the world, including Canada and the US mainly due to the government's reimbursement schemes for the purchase of hardware and software. For, example a GP in the UK can claim up to 50% of expenses for the complete system and in some cases 100% for specific software and training.

In general, the healthcare telematics industry is on the rise mostly in the developed world. While the overall percentage of the healthcare budget spent on information and telecommunication technologies in Europe is relatively low in healthcare (approximately $400 per employee) compared to other sectors such as manufacturing ($1500 per employee) or finance ($5000 per employee) [5]. It is expected to grow due to the new policies and strategies of Member States or due to structural funds provided to some Member States for computerization of healthcare. The expenditure on telematics, presently at a level of 1% on average in Europe of the total health expenditure, is growing with a higher rate than that of investment in telematics in other sectors. In the US it is estimated that the growth of information technologies (IT) expenditure in health sector will reach 15-20% per year [6]. The current European market size for Hospital Information Systems according to Frost & Sullivan is $2.4 Billion compared to $2.7 Billion in United States. Therefore the health telematics industry is on the rise bringing new opportunities for European industry. The Internet, a new generation of mobile services and cards will all find a strong application arena in healthcare.

The figures indicating the overall market of the IT and Telecommunication sectors in the European Union can be found on the web site of EITO – the European Information Technology Observatory (http://www.fvit-eurobit.de/pages/eito/eito002.htm). As we have mentioned before, HII is not the primary force in the development of generic information and telecommunication infrastructure. Therefore, we will not focus on the problems of the generic IT and telecom infrastructure but rather on the particularities of the applications and services that HII would support.

3. Challenges of Wider Implementation

The health sector has not applied information and communication technologies as effectively as have other sectors. Despite the many years of research and development one cannot say that health telematics applications and services are widely used. Also most of the telemedicine services are still under the pilot phase and are usually supported by some research grants. The transfer of research results to practice poses many challenges of various kinds. These challenges can be either related to technological issues or to non-technological issues such as the legal framework, market, vision of decision-makers, and user acceptance issues [7].

In the previous section we have described some of the technological challenges relating to the problems of integration of heterogeneous systems to allow secure and fast communication of patient information that are located in different places (distributed patient record). One could also mention the problems of standardized communications protocols for emergency telemedicine, pattern recognition for automatic analysis of medical images, standardization of the smart card technology to enable the use of health cards across the borders, and the user friendliness of technologies to ensure accessibility and high-quality of interaction for all potential groups of users.

Among the non-technological challenges to implementation it is important to mention the need for a clear legal framework and requirements on the confidentiality of personal data. The European Council and Parliament adopted on October 24th, 1995 a directive on the processing of personal data and free movement of such data (95/46/EC) which needs to be implemented by appropriate national regulations in all Member States by October 24th, 1998. Another challenge is the problem of market fragmentation in Europe. The different legal requirements, different language and specificity of work processes of each country or region lead to the high cost of development and customization. Other relevant directives are the 96/9/EC on the Legal Protection of Databases 97/66/EC - concerning the Processing of Personal Data and the Protection of Privacy in the Telecommunication Sector.

Among the market issues, we can mention the willingness of the industry to invest in good quality products that are based on user requirements. In general the health care market is seen by the industry as large in size but not highly profitable mainly due to lack of standards and high cost of customization. The situation is very fragmented in Europe. For example, most of the countries have a few dozen providers of electronic medical records which have a few installations they cannot communicate with and have difficulties in exporting mainly due to the lack of standards and very different legal requirements. Special industrial activities to tackle these problems are supported by the European Commission in the current R&D Program.

Another important issue is the lack of vision and leadership of the health care managers and health authorities and the lack of willingness to re-engineer the health care processes for the benefits of the quality and efficiency of care delivery. More than half of the Member States have recently adopted strategic plans for using the telematics networks in restructuring the care delivery to support the so-called shared care (managed care) delivery schemes. Some of these plans are described at the web site of European Health Telematics Observatory Project of the Telematics Applications for the Health Sector of the European Commission (http://www.ehto.org).

Finally, the issues of *acceptance and usability* and other human related factors, and the issues of *education and training* are considered to be the most important. Even in the places with the latest technology and the best Intranets the users complain about non-friendliness and speed of the system. Among the many complaints regarding the usability of the system we mention the "lost" time to go to the computer rooms, the speed of retrieving the data, the non-intuitive data input (structured data entry is still not acceptable by most of the physicians), the security procedures (login that takes too much time), the inability of (mobile) interaction with the system while in the corridors or outside of the hospital. The above problems give rise to a series of challenges from the Human-Computer Interaction (HCI) perspective, e.g., intuitive interface metaphors, mobile systems, multimodal interfaces, tailorable and adaptable interfaces, more natural access procedures (e.g. speech interfaces), user identification procedures, and user interfaces for mobile services [8].

4. Conclusions

The new paradigm of citizen-centered shared care is gaining ground in many of the Member States. The information shared by all care providers is patient health-related information, which is comprehensible, reliable and confidential. These information sources will slowly become standardized providing secure access regardless of location and network capacity, scale and security features all the way from fiber optic networks to simple telephone networks and Internet communication. These information sources and networks give rise to Health Information Infrastructure which provides the possibility for rapid dissemination and the sharing of health information and research results, leading to knowledge creation and promotion of innovative approaches based on evidence collected in medical practice all over the world.

This new paradigm is supported by the European Commission in the new Fifth Framework Programme (http://www.cordis.lu). The new proposed program "Creating a User-Friendly Information Society" is split into four key actions. In the first key action "Systems and Services for the Citizens," the proposed activities include creation of the next generation, user-friendly, interoperable and cost-effective services in the areas of health stressing the importance of continuity of care and citizen-centered care. The emphasis will be given in future research and development on accessibility and user-friendliness of telematics applications by applying the theories and technologies of human-computer interaction area. Also, special emphasis will be given to systems for personal health monitoring and prevention, including advanced sensors and micro-systems. Internet health support services to citizens offering health monitoring and prevention services, or between health professionals for teleconsultation and collaborative work, are being set up all over the world.

The global HII requires international collaboration on many of the issues regarding standards and interoperability. The ISO TC215 has been created to tackle the global needs of standardization in health telematics. Finally the new R&D programs of the European Commission have opened up new possibilities for international collaboration with non-EU countries such as Australia, Canada and USA (http://www.cordis.lu).

The views developed in this paper are those of the author and do not necessarily reflect the position of the European Commission.

References

[1] National Committee on Vital and Health Statistics. Assuring a Health Dimension for the National Information Infrastructure, A Concept Paper Presented to the U.S. Department of Health and Human Services Data Council. October 14, 1998, http://aspe.os.dhhs.gov/ncvhs/hii-nii.htm

[2] CPR Attributes and Subattributes. Healthcare Informatics. 1996;13(5):54-62.

[3] J INTERCAM Ltd, Eurotop 13-International results, Aug. 1996 study of the CAM Group, 6 Cantelupe Mews, Cantelupe Road, East Grinstead, Sussex RH19 3BG.

[4] Ahmed, M.A., & Berlin, A. Information Technology in General Practice: current use and views on future development. Journal of Informatics in Primary Care. November 1997.

[5] Bordoni, L. Trends in the European ICT Market, Technical - Report Briefing for the European Commission, International Data Corporation (IDC), March 1996.

[6] Munro, N. "Infotech Reshapes Health Care Marketplace," *Washington Technology*, p.1, Aug. 8, 1996.

[7] Iakovidis, I. "Towards Personal Health Record: Current situation, obstacles and trends in implementation of Electronic Healthcare Records in Europe," *Intern. J. of Medical Informatics*, vol 52, No 123, pg. 105 –117 (1998).

[8] Iakovidis, I. "Interacting with Electronic Healthcare Record in the Information Society," in *Proc. 7th Int. Conf. on Human-Computer Interaction'97*, San Francisco, CA 1997, pp. 811-814.

Information Technology Strategies from
the United States and the European Union
E.A. Balas et al. (Eds)
IOS Press 2000

Interaction Between Clinical Research and Patient Data

Reed M. Gardner, Ph.D.
Professor & Chair, Department of Medical Informatics
University of Utah
Salt Lake City, Utah, USA

1. Introduction

Most computers systems used in hospitals and clinics today are "order entry and charge capture" systems [1]. Despite the fact that many centers have worked at developing clinical information systems, there continues to be a struggle in developing these systems with data acquisition methods, compatibility between systems and transferability of the technology from one institution to another. There is ample evidence from several sources that patients are "harmed" while in the hospital as a result of preventable errors [2,3].

Work that my colleagues and I have done has been principally with the inpatient HELP hospital computer system at LDS Hospital in Salt Lake City, Utah known as HELP [4,5,6]. We are now sharing similar concepts of clinical decision making to the outpatient setting. The concepts I will present are based on practical, clinical applications; I will discuss instrumentation and other methods of gathering and using clinical data for clinical research and patient care.

Gathering patient clinical data is not a trivial problem, even with automation techniques available today in other industries. For example, if we were to gather data only from a ventilator on a patient in a critical care unit, we could gather as much as four megabytes of data per day. Since gathering so much data would overwhelm the usual manual charting systems, gathering it automatically is a bit like receiving "junk mail." We may be collecting data we really do not need, but at times we gather such data, from bedside monitors and the like, just because it is available. Dr. Homer R. Warner had the concept several years ago that we should collect "coded data" into our database, data that would be useful for medical decision-making. By collecting coded clinical data and establishing "knowledge bases" computers could then be used to provide data for review purposes, to generate alerts, to operate protocols etc.

At LDS Hospital in Salt Lake City, we are currently collecting a wide variety of the patient's clinical data and using the data to enhance patient care using the HELP computer system. The highest priority clinical data, in the minds of the clinical staff is laboratory findings. The next most important clinical information would be observational data from nurses and physicians. Then medication records would be of next priority. However, the HELP system has data coming from a wide variety of places, simple data that you would think would not be terribly important for clinical things until you think about it. For example, the surgery schedule turns out to be a very important driver for preventing deep venous thrombosis as well as helping to prevent post-operative wound infections.

When we started developing the HELP system, there were no standard coding systems, as a consequence, we had to develop our own. At this point in the development of enterprise wide information systems, we would love to have a common coding system that we could share among the 23 hospitals in our own health care enterprise, with hospitals in Salt Lake City, across the United States, and eventually with health care facilities throughout the world. Developing such standards is a huge problem that needs to be solved and international cooperation would be a tremendous assistance.

Figure 1 is a block diagram of the HELP system. For example if we have a life-threatening Serum Potassium value of 6.2. The data flows into the database and the HELP system "data drives" and activates the knowledge base. The knowledge base has a rule that triggers when the Potassium is above 6.0 and causes an alert to be generated [7]. The nurse caring for that particular patient is paged. Recently, investigators at Brigham and Women's Hospital have improved on the strategy, they page the medical Resident caring for the patient [8]. Both teams have shown that response times to patient care have been reduced from several hours to several minutes.

At each bedside at LDS Hospital, not only the ICU beds, there is a bedside computer terminal, conveniently located such that nurses, physicians, and other care givers can enter data and review data. Much of the data from bedside devices, such as monitors, is automatically collected. However, nurses provide a major part of the clinical data input. Physicians do mostly data review and they love it. I have a son who just recently received his medical degree. When he came to LDS Hospital and used the computer, he said, "Dad, it's like practicing medicine at the country club. You can go 20 minutes before rounds and

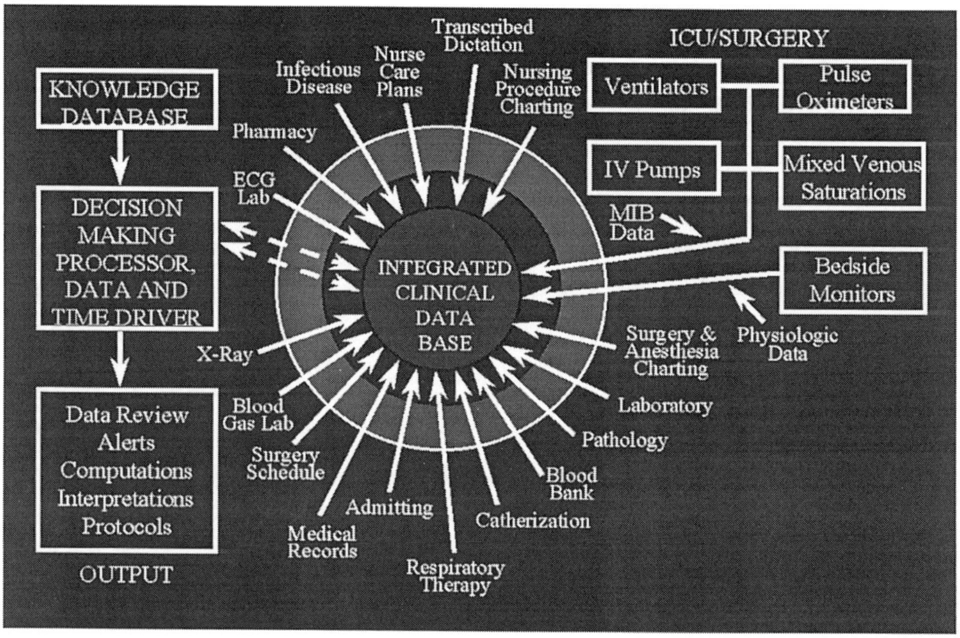

Figure 1: HELP System

be prepared, whereas if you go to the University and VA hospital, you aren't prepared after spending two hours." The HELP system provides a variety of methods of reviewing patient data which physicians appreciate.

As shown in Figure 1, bedside monitors, the IV pumps and other devices are connected through a Medical Information Bus interface [9,10]. We have found that human observers are not perfect data collectors. In most hospitals, vital sign and other information is taken from bedside monitors and written on a large flow sheet. We have found that many times, even in critical care physician order vital signs on a "Q two hours" basis. For some reason nurses interpret that to mean that the measures must be taken exactly on the hour. For example, I have seen nurses come to the bedside at 30 to 45 minutes past the hour, view the bedside monitor and chart the result as having occurred on the hour. After having observed such behavior, I have asked the nurses why? I get a response such as "Well, the physician expects the results to be recorded within a minute or two of the hour." As a result, there are large "timing" as well as data collection errors.

Medicine is really inherently an information science. The better knowledge and information that is available to clinicians, the better they can diagnose, counsel and advise their patients. Also, the better treatment they can give and as a consequence better outcomes can be achieved.

There are still fundamental data collection questions that must be resolved. For example: Who should supply the data? What patient data are needed? How frequently are the data needed? What methods (automatic, manual) should be used to collect the data? How reliable are the data that are being collected?

To deal with a few of these questions such as "Who supplies the data?" At the LDS Hospital, the nurses provide most of the observational data, and the physicians provide some. "What data are needed?" Every health care system need to identify a patient. We have a serious problem in the United States right now; we would like to have a common identifier. However, we have not been able to achieve such a standard because of concerns about privacy and confidentiality and do not currently have adequate rules (laws) about how to handle the privacy and confidentiality issues of computerized patient records. Someone asked me the other day how many places privacy was mentioned in the United States Constitution. The U.S. Constitution is indeed a remarkable document, but privacy is never mentioned. It is my understanding that Europeans have workable public policies on privacy. Recently, in the United States there has been a suggestion that patients be given the right to prevent any of their record from being entered into a computer. If a patient came to our facility, we would have to say "I'm sorry we can't care for you because virtually every monitoring and laboratory instrument in our hospital has a computer in it."

Other data that must be collected is demographic data, diagnostic codes, and a wide variety of clinical data, and charge and "cost" data. I am fortunate to work at a corporation that actually knows what each procedure, medication etc costs. We know what the medication costs as well as knowing what it costs for the nurse to give the medication. Short term data from hospitalization is available in our system. However, long-term (months to years after hospital treatment are not known).

"How frequently should patient data be collected?" Clearly it makes a difference if the patient is in a critical care unit versus is receiving "home care" with weekly visits from a care provider. However, it would be good to have rules and strategies about how frequently data should be collected. It is my feeling that only by developing computerized databases can we begin to answer this question.

"What methods (automatic, manual) should be used to collect the data?" Gathering data from automated instruments is the ideal data collection strategy. I have had nurses comment to me, "Dr. Gardner, we know enough about computers. And we know what you can do with them. We don't ever want to read data from one computer screen and enter it into another computer." Perhaps, an even worse scenario is to have the nurse read data from a computer screen and write it down on a piece of paper, then at a later time have the data abstracted by manual chart review!

"How reliable are the data that are being collected?" Virtually every experiment we have done shows that data collected with the discipline required by "coding" and "computer entry" are more reliable than data collected by manually abstracting records from paper charts.

Nurses, physicians, and medical records staff provide codes for diagnoses and procedures performed. As already mentioned, most computers used in hospitals today are for billing and accounting purposes. We must change the paradigm of data collection. We must collect clinical data for clinical purposes and as a "by product" derive the charging and billing information.

How are data currently collected in most health care systems? Unfortunately, most data for studies is done by "manual chart review." We pay a nurse or another care provider to do manual chart review. Wouldn't it be wonderful if we had a computer-based record? We cold then review the computer records promptly and efficiently and minimize cost of data abstraction and collection. Manual chart review is very inefficient, it is very expensive, it is not "real time" and the accuracy is poor.

What are the advantages of computer records? They can be real time, they have excellent accuracy, we can control what data is collected, and we can have computerized decision support. As a consequence, we should all be promoting computerized clinical records.

What are the problems? Computerized records are very difficult to establish because of a huge initial investment both in terms of money and people training. After installing computerized records systems, it takes at least two years before you can expect any outcomes. In the United States, we as a people seem to want everything quickly. Administrators, physicians and other clinicians seem to think that all that must be done is to install a bunch of PCs and "magically" you will have a patient record system.

Realistically if you install a clinical computing system in a 500 bed hospital, you will likely spend at least $10,000,000 dollars for hardware and software system, and another $10,000,000 to train the clinical staff. If you can not show exciting results by the fourth or fifth year, do not give up. It may take you six or seven years. Installing computerized records system requires huge cultural and process changes. "Change experts" tell me that change is not easy.

How reliable are data? In our experience, if data are clinically relevant they are more reliable. If the data are used for clinical decision making, they are usually reliable. Financial data, if it is used for management purposes is quite reliable. However, we still get "composite data" from our corporate office that is clearly in error. As a result we must go through and "clean the data."

Dr. Clement C. McDonald, who is one of our good informatics colleagues has said "When it comes to gathering information, medicine hasn't evolved much from the hunting and gathering stages of social evolution." Recently, a graduate student in our department looked at data across the health care enterprise and found that asking even simple questions such as "How many Catholics do we serve?" were impossible to answer because of a large variety of coding methods. Even more absurd was that fact that establishing a standard for "gender" was problematic.

In medicine, we think we have unique problems when it comes to gathering patient data. Such is not the case. A recent IEEE Computer publication illustrates the general nature of computerized data capture with their article was entitled "10 Potholes in the Road to Information Quality" [11]. Potholes are the little holes that develop in highways that quickly grow and become hazardous to automobile travel. Four of the "potholes" related to medical computing were: 1) Multiple sources of the same information produces different values. For example: When a hospital uses two separate methods to assess severity of illness; 2) Information is produced using subjective judgements leading to bias. For example: When medical coders use their independent judgement to select disease codes; 3) Systematic errors in information production lead to lost information. For example: Information was missed because an edit check would not be accepted (such as not allowing a weight over 150 kg when the patient's actual weight was 160 kg); 4) Distributed heterogeneous systems lead to inconsistent definitions, formats, and values. For example: Different systems in each hospital may use different formats for diagnostic codes.

2. Practical Examples of Use of Computers and Data in Clinical Medicine

Let me share with you some work that Scott Evans, David Classin, John Burke, and Stan Postotnik have done at LDS Hospital using computers to improve antibiotics use [12,13,14,15,16,17]. First, you must understand that antibiotics are a very effective method to treat infections, but they can also cause health care problems such as: 1) Increase patient mortality and morbidity; 2) Cause adverse drug events (ADE); 3) Increase bacterial resistance by overuse, and 4) Increase hospital costs since antibiotics are among the most expensive medications used in hospitals.

To answer the question "What is the cost of a surgical infection?" these investigators used archived HELP system computer records to match patients who had infections with those who did not [12]. Using the archived records and the "cost" data available in the integrated accounting system, they were able to match patients by disease, age, etc. They were able to answer the following questions about a patient who had hospital acquired infections:

- What was the attributable cost of a hospital acquired infection? It was $4,935.
- What was the attributable increase in length of stay? It was 5.34 days.
- What was the attributable increase in mortality rate? Mortality rate increased from 1.12% to 6.80% if the patient had an infection.

Although animals studies had given an indication as to when the best time to give antibiotics before surgery in humans. This group "mined" the clinical database from the HELP system and asked "When is the best time to give a prophylactic antibiotic for a patient going to surgery?" [13]. They found that giving the prophylactic too soon, more than two hours before the surgery, and too late, after the surgery begins lead to higher infection rates. As a result they determined that a two hour window before surgery was the optimum time. A careful review of patient records showed that only about 40% of patients needing prophylactic antibiotics were receiving them in the two hour time window. In addition, they found that many patients were receiving their prophylactic antibiotics for a period far too long after the surgery. If these situations could be corrected, prophylactic antibiotics would be more effective, and costs of antibiotics could be decreased.

To improve the frequency of "appropriate prophylaxis" a simple "ABX" was inserted onto the computer generated surgical schedule. In addition, educational sessions about optimal post operative antibiotic administration duration were conducted [14]. The result was a dramatic improvement prophylactic antibiotics given in the two hour time window before surgery (appropriateness of administration and timing increased to 99%). In addition for the period from 1985 to 1993 the number of post operative antibiotic doses per patient decreased from 19 per patient to only 6 per patient resulting in an estimated annual savings of $324,000.

During the early phases of the project, physicians asked: "What if we choose not to give prophylactic antibiotics and the computer has recommended them? Then if that particular patient got an infection, wouldn't we get sued?" To help answer this question, a "natural experiment" occurred. The program that printed the ABX notifier on the surgery schedule was inoperative for a time. During this time interval the prophylaxis rate decreased to 70%. Based on this finding, LDS Hospital's Medical Executive Committee decided to keep the ABX on the surgery schedule because of the important improvement in prophylaxis and decrease that had been seen in post operative infections. In the decade since that decision no one has been sued.

In a parallel study looking at antibiotic management at LDS Hospital during 1988 and during 1994, the following exciting results were found [14]. In 1988, the antibiotic cost per patient was $123 and in 1994 it was only $52. Total pharmacy medications costs for 1988 were $3,980,00 and in 1994 $4,760,000. The antibiotics cost in 1988 were $990,000 or 25% of the total medications cost. However, in 1994, the antibiotic costs were only $610,000 or 13% of the total medications cost. In addition there was a higher severity of illness (case mix index) in 1994 than in 1988. More wide-spectrum antibiotics were used in 1994 (47%) versus 24% in 1988. There was no change in the pattern of resistant bacteria between the two periods. LDS Hospital maintained an "open" drug formulary, that is the improvement was not made by restricting use of new and very expensive antibiotics. Overall antibiotic use decreased by 23%. Hospital mortality rate decreased from 3.65 to 2.65%. Antibiotics cost per patient decreased by 42%. Finally there was a 30% reduction in antibiotics-associated Adverse Drug Events from 1988 to 1994.

3. Adverse Drug Events

Investigators at LDS Hospital conducted "So what?" studies [15,16,17]. During a 12 month period from May 1988 through April 1989 there were 9 adverse drug events (ADE) recorded for 25,142 admissions (rate 0.04%). However, they had a feeling that the true number of events was not being recorded. Then the investigators began looking, using the computer record as a tool, at when patients got antidotes reviewing nursing notes for and other evidence of an adverse drug event. They found that the real ADE rate was about 2.3%! It was a bit like if I were driving from here (Columbia, Missouri) to St. Louis, Missouri and I looked down at the speedometer and was going 90 miles per hour, well over the 65 mile per hour speed limit. Would you drive off the freeway at the next town and find the sheriff or the highway patrolman? I wouldn't. A similar process was in effect with the caregivers. If there was an Adverse Drug Event and they could promptly and properly treat the event, the event was apparently never recorded. However, having the computer monitor such events, in its tireless way, then the important events that required monitoring could be easily and promptly followed up on. If you find an ADE, you can respond to them quickly and it really makes a difference.

Using methodologies similar to those used to detect the detrimental effects of infections, Medical Informatics students used the HELP database and determined the following detrimental effects of ADEs. The hospital cost attributable to an ADE was $1,939. The increased length of stay was 1.94 days and the mortality increased from 1.05% to 3.50% for matched cohorts of patients [17]. Other investigators have used similar computer methods to prevent serious medication errors [18].

4. Computerized Antibiotic Assistant

At LDS Hospital, if a physician wishes to order antibiotics, they go to the bedside computer terminal and select the "antibiotic assistant" option. A computerized antibiotic assistant was initially developed for the Shock-Trauma Intensive Care Unit. Physicians in this ICU treat some of the most difficult trauma and surgical patients at LDS Hospital. These physicians had experience with computerized "protocols" for management of patients with Adult Respiratory Distress Syndrome (ARDS) and felt that computerized decision support would be helpful in suggesting antibiotic therapy.

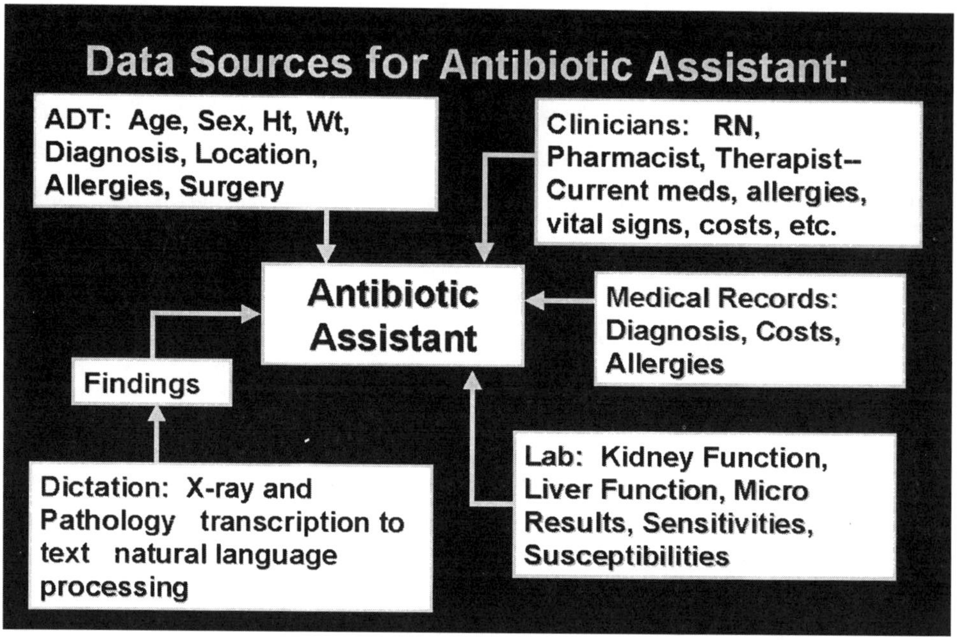

Figure 2: Data Sources for Antibiotic Assistant

In a recent publication in *The New England Journal of Medicine*, Scott Evans and his colleagues outline the development and evaluation of the computerized "antibiotic assistant" [19]. The computer uses data from a wide variety of sources that are stored in its integrated database to assist the physician in ordering antibiotics. Figure 2 shows a simplified diagram of the data sources and how they are integrated into the HELP system so that computerized decision-support rules can be applied.

Figure 3 shows the display that appears on the screen for a 43 year old patient in the Shock-Trauma Intensive Care Unit, with Adult Respiratory Distress Syndrome (ARDS). The patient's maximum white blood count (WBC) for the past 24 hours is 12.7 an increase from 11.7 the day before. Patient temperature is 38.1 C a decrease from 38.5 C the day before. Renal function as determined by the laboratory results shown is decreased. The patient is allergic to penicillins. The patient is currently on Nystatin with the dose shown. Displayed on the next lines are the pathogens identified for sputum and a urinary catheter. Next are the computer recommendations for this specific patient. Note that the current medication and the recommendations are different. If the physician chose to use the 3 antibiotics shown, all they would be required to do is press the "*" key and "Return." If they wanted to have the computer "Explain" why it has made the recommendations pressing a “4" and then “Return” would provide the reasons. One of the reasons for this patient was “Positive respiratory culture that was supported by a chest X-ray of 9/13.” The computer system takes the dictation produced by the radiologist and uses natural language processing to determine if there is evidence from the dictation to indicate pneumonia. The natural language processing has an accuracy of 90%, and is not perfect, but having any data from the chest X-ray is certainly better than having no data. A similar natural language program evaluates relevant pathology dictation information.

Forty-six percent of the orders were followed. It is better than that, but it is still not perfect. Ninety-three percent of the doses in intervals were followed. The clinicians can choose another antibiotic and it will get better. The computerized antibiotic assistant:

- Took about 4 seconds to gather data which it takes a human about 15 minutes to collect
- Antibiotic allergies decreased from 13% to 6%
- Adverse Drug Events due to antibiotic uses decreased from 2.5% to 0.7%
- Excess doses decreased from 36% to 16%
- Mismatches between finding from the microbiological laboratory susceptibilities decreased from 18% to 2%
- Excess time on the antibiotic was decreased from 5.9 to 2.7 days
- Cost of antibiotics decreased from $427 to $102 per patient

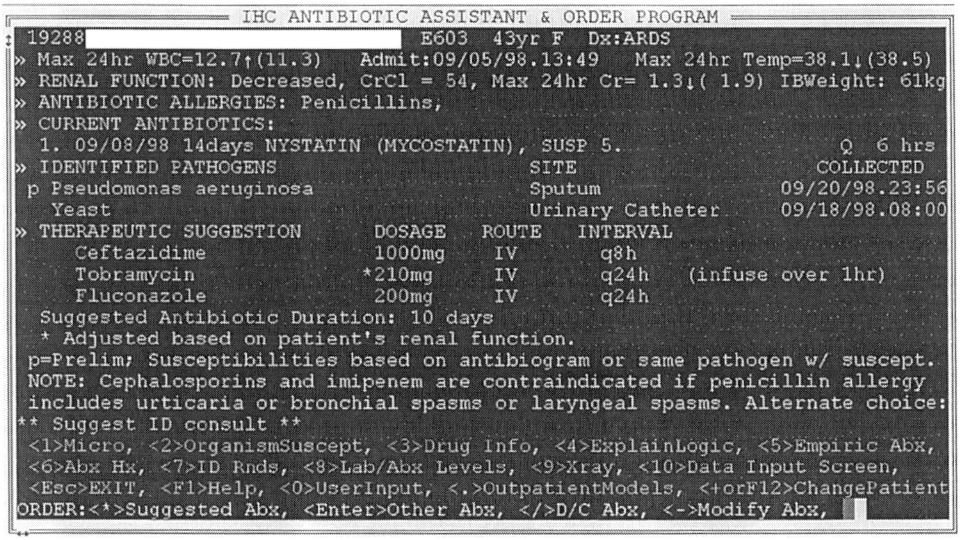

Figure 3: Display Screen for Antibiotic Assistant

- Hospital length of stay for matched patients decreased from 16.7 to 10.0 days when the computer recommendation was followed
- Total hospital costs were dramatically reduced

The antibiotic assistant has been so successful that it is now used hospital wide and in fact is being used at several of Intermountain Health Care's larger hospital facilities. In conclusion, from the materials presented above it is clear that:

1. Computerized record systems are a valuable tool in optimizing medical care.
2. Integration of cost and clinical data provides a powerful tool for doing cost/benefit analysis.
3. Integrated clinical computing systems are practical and useful to physicians and other care givers.
4. Clinical computing systems can be used to reduce inappropriate use of antibiotics, and in fact can suggest the "best" antibiotic regimen.
5. The number of adverse drug events can be minimized and the deleterious effects of ADE's minimized by using computers to detect and act on these events promptly.
6. Preliminary views of Cost and Benefit of clinical computing systems are encouraging.

References

[1] Kleinke, J.D. Release 0.0: Clinical information technology in the real world. Health Affairs (Millwood). 1998;17(6):23-38.

[2] Leape, L.L. Error in medicine. JAMA: The Journal of the American Medical Medical Association. 1994;272(23):1851-1857.

[3] Leape, L.L., Woods, D.D., Hatlie, M.J., Kizer, K.W., & Schroeder, S.A., Lundberg GD. Promoting patient safety by preventing medical error. JAMA: The Journal of the American Medical Association. 1998;280(16):1444-1447.

[4] Kuperman, G.J., Gardner, R.M., & Pryor, T.A. HELP: A Dynamic Hospital Information System. Springer-Verlag Inc, New York, NY 1991.

[5] Grandia, L.C., Pryor, T.A., & Willson, D.F. et al. Building a Computer-based Patient Record System in an Evolving Integrated Health System. First Annual Nicholas E. Davies CPR Recognition Symposium Proceedings, Edited by Elaine B. Steen. Pages 3 to 33. April 4-6, 1995. {Republished in 1999 by McGraw Hill for the Computerized Record Institute (CPRI)}

[6] Gardner, R.M., Pryor, T.A., & Warner, H.R. The HELP System: Functionality Update. International Journal of Medical Informatics (In Press)

[7] Tate, K.E., Gardner, R.M., & Scherting, K. Nurses, Pagers, and Patient-Specific Criteria: Three Keys to Improved Critical Value Reporting. Journal of the American Medical Informatics Association 1995; 2(symposium supplement):164-168.

[8] Kuperman, G.J., Boyle, D., Jha, A., et al. How promptly are inpatients treated for critical laboratory results? Journal of the American Medical Informatics Association. 1998;5(1):112-119.

[9] Kennelly, R.J., Gardner, R.M. Perspectives on development of IEEE 1073: The Medical Information Bus (MIB) Standard. International Journal of Clinical Monitoring & Computing 1997: 14:143-149.

[10] Dalto JS, Johnson KV, Gardner RM, Spuhler VJ, Egbert L. Medical Information Bus usage for automated IV pump data acquisition: Evaluation of use and nurse attitudes. International Journal of Clinical Monitoring & Computing 1997;14:151-154

[11] Strong, D.M., Lee, Y.W., & Wang, R.Y. 10 potholes in the road to information quality. IEEE Computer 1997;30(8):38-46.

[12] Classen DC. Assessing the Effect of Adverse Hospital Events on the Cost of Hospitalization and Other Patient Outcomes. MS Thesis in Medical Informatics, University of Utah 1993.

[13] Classen, D.C., Evans, R.S., Pestotnik, S.L., Horn, S.D., Menlove, R.L. & Burke, J.P. The timing of prophylactic administration of antibiotics and the risk of surgical-wound infection. New England Journal of Medicine. 1992;326(5):281-286.

[14] Pestotnik, S.L., Classen, D.C., Evans, R.S., & Burke, J.P. Implementing antibiotic practice guidelines through computer-assisted decision support: clinical and financial outcomes. Annals of Internal Medicine. 1996;124(10):884-890.

[15] Evans RS, Classen DC, Stevens LE, Pestotnik SL, et al. Using a hospital information system to assess the effects of adverse drug events. Proceedings of the Annual Symposium on Computer Applications in Medical Care. 1993;161-165.

[16] Evans RS, Pestotnik SL, Classen DC, Horn SD, Bass SB and Burke JP. Preventing adverse drug events in hospitalized patients. Annals of Pharmacotherapy. 1994;28(4):523-527.

[17] Classen, D.C., Pestotnik, S.L., Evans, R.S., Lloyd, J.F., & Burke, J.P. Adverse drug events in hospitalized patients. Excess length of stay, extra costs, and attributable mortality. JAMA: The Journal of the American Medical Association. 1997;277(4):301-306.

[18] Bates, D.W., Leape, L.L., Cullen, D.J., Laird, N., Peterson, L.A., & Teich, J.M. Effect of computerized physician order entry and a team intervention on prevention of serious medication errors. JAMA: The Journal of the American Medical Association. 1998;280(15):1311-1316.

[19] Evans RS, Pestotnik SL, Classen DC, et al. A computer-assisted management program for antibiotics and other antiinfective agents. New England Journal of Medicine. 1998;338(4):232-238.

Structuring Knowledge for Practical Application

Information Technology Strategies from the United States and the European Union
E.A. Balas et al. (Eds)
IOS Press 2000

Digital Library Research and Application

Alexa T. McCray, Ph.D.
Director, Lister Hill National Center for Biomedical Communications
National Library of Medicine
Bethesda, Maryland, USA

Abstract. The last decade has seen an exponential rise in the amount and the nature of information that is available on the Internet. Internet and World Wide Web technology have raised many technical as well as social and economic issues. The paper begins with a description of the recent digital library research initiative funded by the U.S. federal government. Digital library research addresses a host of informatics issues relevant to the current Internet-based environment. The paper continues with a discussion of some problems in information access, including a discussion of the potential of the Unified Medical Language System for navigating among multiple biomedical information systems. Next, some issues in creating Web-accessible resources for health care consumers are addressed, with a focus on recent work at the National Library of Medicine, including a description of the MEDLINE*plus* system. The paper ends with a brief discussion of some implications of digital library research for the health informatics community.

1. Introduction

The last decade has seen an exponential rise in the amount and the nature of information that is available on the Internet. A 1998 report from the National Coordination Office for Computing, Information and Communications states that the Internet has grown at nearly 100% per year since 1988, and that Internet traffic has been growing at 400% per year (http://www.ccic.gov/ngi/implementation). World Wide Web technology has made it possible to search and deliver large amounts of digital information at incredible speed anywhere in the world at any time. People from all walks of life are using the Web for all sorts of tasks. They read the news online; they shop; they play the stock market; and they check the movie listings for their favorite theaters. High school students use the Web to complete homework assignments, and serious researchers find that many of their regular journals have come online. Increasingly, patients and their families are using the Web to research their health problems, searching, sometimes in vain, for relevant, accurate and timely information about the diagnosis or treatment of their disease.

The technology provides tremendous opportunities, but it does not come without some cost. The sheer volume of material on the Web often makes it difficult to find the information wanted, and its highly variable quality can pose serious problems, particularly in an area as important as health care. Lagoze and Fielding summarize the characteristics of the Web as follows: "The World Wide Web provides unprecedented access to globally distributed content. The success of the Web, both in terms of number of resources and use of those resources, is largely due to three defining characteristics... Because of its universality, anyone can participate in the Web, as author, publisher, or consumer, with a minimal investment of hardware and expertise. Because of its uniformity, resources, and services, users participate on the Web as equals in a common information space. Finally, because of decentralization, the Web is fundamentally anarchistic beyond basic agreement at the technical level on protocols and transport mechanisms" [1].

The following touches on some of the issues that have been raised by World Wide Web technology and use. It begins by describing digital library research, which addresses a host of informatics issues relevant to the current Internet-based environment. It continues by discussing, in somewhat greater detail, problems in information access, indicating that the Unified Medical Language System (UMLS) project might be seen as a type of semantic "middleware" for navigating among multiple biomedical information systems. Next it addresses some issues in creating Web-accessible resources for health care consumers, focusing on recent work at the National Library of Medicine (NLM), including the MEDLINE*plus* system. It ends by considering some implications of digital library research for the health informatics community.

2. Digital Library Research

The term "digital library" has been coined to refer to Internet accessible collections of digital information, and digital library research has become an active area of investigation in the last several years. The U.S. Federal government has been a catalyst in this research by funding a significant amount of work through its Digital Library Initiative [2,3]. The National Library of Medicine's involvement in the second phase of this initiative has helped expand the pool of researchers involved in digital library research to the health and medical informatics community. A wide range of issues is addressed in the digital library research agenda, encompassing three broad areas of research: human-centered research, content and collections-based research, and systems-centered research.

Human-centered research is concerned with methods to improve access to information, including retrieval algorithms, filtering methods, and user interface design. With the wealth of information already available on the Internet, and with the expectation that it will continue to grow unabated, new methods are needed to organize, link, and filter information resources for specialized audiences and purposes. Users are confronted with a sometimes bewildering array of available information and have few tools to manage, sort, and assess the quality of the information that is presented to them. Current Web search engines, though seemingly quite powerful, are nonetheless limited in their ability to effectively index, retrieve, and rank the information they find across the wide range of distributed resources available on the Internet. The engines use different methods and algorithms for indexing Web resources and for ranking the retrieval results; they differ in the frequency with which they capture data on the Web; and they return widely differing retrieval sets given the same query. Lynch points out that the Web has "evolved into what might be thought of as a chaotic repository for the collective output of the world's printing presses", and that what will be needed is a combination of the librarian's classification skills and the computer scientist's ability to automate indexing and searching processes [4].

Content and collections-based research involves the technical, social, and economic issues related to the creation and management of digital collections. For conversion projects decisions need to be made about the optimal scanning resolution and the robustness of the optical character recognition technology (OCR) used. Often, particularly for older, faded, or otherwise inferior original documents, the OCR is inadequate. For these cases as well as for digital photos, audio, and video, the metadata that describes the digital object is the only reliable way to search for and access that item. Whether digital resources are "born digitally" or are converted to electronic form by scanning technology, serious issues arise when considering their persistence over long periods of time [5]. It is important to consider whether an organization has the resources to ensure the ongoing preservation and inevitable conversion of digital materials from one medium to another that will be required when software and hardware change over time, and whether the organization is willing to make that commitment [6,7]. Much of the material that is "published" on the Web is freely available, and many are beginning to question the constraints that traditional copyright imposes on the distribution of information. Publishers, authors, and libraries all have a role to play in the resolution of these thorny intellectual property rights issues. There seems to be little doubt that new economic models for distributing Internet-based information will evolve.

Systems-centered research includes the development of core digital library technologies, including system scalability, open, networked architectures, and reusable, standard tools. The robustness of the Internet infrastructure itself is of concern, particularly for sophisticated image-intensive applications, such as many medical and scientific applications, that require high-speed lines and extensive bandwidth. Improved methods are needed for accessing the highly distributed data that often only resides in the so-called "hidden tier" of back-end databases [8]. Real-time simultaneous searching of large numbers of distributed databases will require basic research in federated database technology. Methods for evaluating the performance of Internet applications are needed. While it is important for information providers to know how well they are serving their intended audiences, few evaluation measures exist and little formal evaluation is being conducted.

3. Information Access

There is a rich history of information retrieval research, which has been primarily concerned with retrieval methods and algorithms [9]. An information space that is as large and complex as today's growing Internet will, however, require new models for effective searching, browsing, and display. Lawrence and Giles analyzed the capabilities of six well-known Internet search engines and found that the coverage of any single engine was quite limited, with none of them indexing more than about one-third of the resources that were actually available on the Web at the time of the study [10]. As a simple experiment, one could submit the term "fibromyalgia" to four different search engines. "Fibroyalgia" is significant because it was one of the most frequently searched terms on the NLM home page during a recent three month period. There were significant differences in the number of items returned from the four engines. AltaVista returned 88,291 items; Excite returned 13,447; Google returned 4,166; and Yahoo, after choosing the health category, returned 68 items. The Excite engine returned a definition for fibromyalgia together with links to symptoms, treatment, and prevention, before listing its other hits. Altavista questioned the spelling, and then listed several related searches, including "fibromyalgia syndrome", "fibromyalgia treatment", and "fibromyalgia support group", also before listing its other hits. A comparison of the top ten items returned by each of the engines showed very little overlap. AltaVista and Google had two items in common, though they were ranked differently.

The difficulties associated with resource discovery have led to a variety of proposals for describing information resources on the Web [11]. Metadata systems have been devised that describe digital documents and other digital objects. In addition to basic information, such as the title, author, and source and date of publication, metadata may also include a description of the content of the document, index terms from a controlled vocabulary, and links to related documents. Information providers are slowly beginning to incorporate metadata in the documents they publish on the Web, and several search engines are giving higher ranking priority to structured metadata information. The NLM's *Profiles in Science* project involves the digital conversion of archival materials, and has a metadata system at the core of its system's architecture [12]. The project is making the collections of prominent biomedical scientists available on the World Wide Web (http://profiles.nlm.nih.gov/). The collections have been donated to the NLM and contain published and unpublished materials, including books, journal articles, diaries, letters, electronic files, photographs, audio tapes, and other audiovisual materials. The initial collection on the site represents the work of Oswald T. Avery, one of the first molecular biologists, whose findings proved that the genetic material is DNA. The second collection represents the work of Joshua Lederberg who received the Nobel Prize for his discoveries concerning genetic recombination and the organization of the genetic material of bacteria. Additional collections will be added regularly.

Even when their creators have explicitly described digital resources, successful mapping of users' queries to information resources still remains a serious challenge. Often this is because there is a mismatch between the way the user has expressed a concept and the way in which that same concept is represented in the information resource. As Brooks has pointed out "...language itself is the fundamental problem of IR [information retrieval]... Construction of large IR systems without more regard to fundamental language problems will inevitably result in the construction of electronic Towers of Babel" [13]. The development of tools to mediate between the language of users and the information sources they attempt to access has been the primary objective of the NLM's UMLS project. The UMLS knowledge sources have been released annually since 1990 for use in informatics research and applications, and, as a consequence, have benefited from collaboration with researchers from all over the world. In 1999 over 1,000 individuals or institutions signed the UMLS license agreement and some 700 of these are accessing the UMLS data through the Internet-based UMLS Knowledge Source Server (http://umlsks.nlm.nih.gov/) [14].

The January 1998 issue of the Journal of the American Medical Informatics Association was devoted to a review of some of the work that has been done in the project since its beginnings [15,16,17,18,19,20,21]. The most extensive of the UMLS knowledge sources is the Metathesaurus. The Metathesaurus integrates and interrelates a variety of existing terminologies. The 1999 version of the Metathesaurus contains over 600,000 biomedical concepts with more than a million different names interrelating some 40 source vocabularies. The terminologies cover a wide spectrum of health care concerns, including broad terminologies, such as SNOMED and MeSH, and more specific terminologies encompassing cancer, psychiatry, radiology, dentistry, epidemiology, nursing, and many other areas. Translations for portions of the UMLS terminologies are available in several languages, including German, French, Spanish, Portuguese, Italian, Norwegian, Swedish, Finnish, and Hungarian. The semantic network, through its 134 semantic types and 54 relations gives semantic coherence to the Metathesaurus and all of its disparate terminologies. Semantic types are assigned to each concept in the Metathesaurus, allowing users and computerized systems to categorize and relate the concepts to each other. The third knowledge source comprises the SPECIALIST lexicon and its associated lexical tools. All three knowledge sources can be used by applications in such a way that users are protected from the myriad language variations that are often significant stumbling blocks as users attempt to access biomedical information.

As electronic patient record systems are becoming a reality, there has been even greater recognition of the need for a robust clinical terminology. The Large Scale Vocabulary Test was conducted in 1996 to help answer the question, "To what extent does the clinical terminology that we need already exist?" [22]. We designed a fully Internet-based experiment that involved 63 participants from around the country who submitted over 40,000 terms to the UMLS. Fifty-eight percent of the terms mapped directly to already existing terminologies in the Metathesaurus. Another 41 percent were related in some way to terms in the existing terminologies. In two thirds of these latter cases, the user's term was narrower in meaning than the concept that already exists. The results of the test showed that while no individual vocabulary was sufficient to represent the terminology that is needed for electronic patient records and other clinical applications, a combination of existing controlled vocabularies does represent the meanings of the majority of the terminology needed for such applications.

Although UMLS research began well before the recent explosion of Internet-based resources, its primary goal has always been to provide tools for navigating among disparate sources of information. The UMLS knowledge sources might, thus, usefully be viewed as semantic "middleware" that can be used in applications for improved access to biomedical information. The concept of middleware has been defined in the computer science literature to refer to services that run at the interface between specific computer platforms and the higher level applications with which users interact [23]. Middleware services are general purpose services that meet the needs of a variety of applications and that both support and promote standard protocols for the exchange of information. An example of using the UMLS as middleware in an Internet search engine is the Medical World Search system (http://mwsearch.com/), which is specifically designed to find high quality medical information on the Internet [24].

4. Creating Web-accessible Resources

Early examples of projects that created Web-based medical resources specifically for patients as well as health care professionals include the University of Iowa's Virtual Hospital and Oncolink from the University of Pennsylvania, though there were several others as well [25,26,27]. The last few years have seen a dramatic increase in the number of patients who are searching for health information on the World Wide Web. They may be searching the Web just to get a basic understanding of what their disease is, or to get information on the latest treatments, or to find support groups or organizations that specialize in their disease. Bader and Braude, in a recent article, suggest that patient access to Internet information will undoubtedly have a significant impact on the relationship between physicians and their patients [28]. They recommend that medical schools take the lead in several areas, including creating high quality electronic resources, joining with libraries to organize and evaluate existing Web resources, and adding courses in "patient informatics" to the medical school curriculum, so that the practitioners of tomorrow are better able to respond to their patients. Bader and Braude, only partly in jest, suggest that the traditional history and physical might be expanded to include not only questions such as

"What medications are you taking?" but also, perhaps, "What Internet sites have you visited?"

Many Web sites have been developed with the health care consumer in mind; so many, in fact, patients are warned to be cautious and to evaluate a site carefully. In October 1998, the Journal of the American Medical Association (JAMA), for example, on its featured "Patient Page" made suggestions designed to help patients determine the quality of online health information [29]. The editors recommend that patients check the source and funding of a site, warning that information that seems primarily to promote a product or position, or that touts "miracle cures" is not to be trusted. They note that the update frequency of the site, who is responsible for reviewing the accuracy of the information, and the listing of the authors' affiliations and credentials are all important indicators of the reliability of a site.

NLM's MEDLINE*plus* lists many resources to assist patients and their families to locate authoritative health information, and uses guidelines to select appropriate sources of health care information (http://www.nlm.nih.gov/medlineplus/). The guidelines are used to assess the quality, authority, and accuracy of content, including the source of the content, the appropriateness of the material to the intended audience, and the quality of any additional links on the site. The consistent availability and frequent updating of the site are also important criteria. The site should be freely available, and its purpose should be primarily to educate and not to sell a product or service.

MEDLINE*plus* provides a range of information intended for health care consumers. Links to directories of health care professionals and facilities, major national organizations providing consumer information, clearinghouses, and libraries are all included. For example, U.S. government consumer health publications from the Centers for Disease Control and Prevention, the National Institutes of Health, and the Food and Drug Administration are available. Online resources such as the Atlas of the Human Body and the Iowa Health Book are featured, as are several online news sources, including health news from the ABC television network, health news from major newspapers such as the New York Times and USA Today, and the JAMA Patient Page. MEDLINE*plus* also links to several dictionaries and glossaries; for example, the Merriam Webster Medical Dictionary, CancerWeb's online medical dictionary, the PharmInfoNet glossary, a glossary prepared by the NIH Office of Rare Diseases, and a multilingual glossary whose creation was sponsored by the European Commission several years ago. This glossary is interesting because it includes not only technical medical terms but also popular terms (http://allserv.rug.ac.be/~rvdstich/eugloss/welcome.html). The glossary includes some 1800 medical terms in nine languages: English, Danish, German, Spanish, French, Italian, Dutch, Portuguese, and Greek.

The most extensive feature of the MEDLINE*plus* site is its health topics, which currently number about 200. Many common diseases and conditions, as well some nutritional and prevention topics are included. For each topic, links are made to diagnosis, treatment, clinical trials, basic research, and organizations that specialize in the topic. For example, for Alzheimer's disease, links are made to several organizations, including the National Institute of Neurological Disorders and Stroke, the National Institute of Mental Health, the National Institute on Aging, the Alzheimer's Association, and the Alzheimer's Disease Education and Referral Center. In addition, for this topic, links are made to several groups that help family members and others cope with caring for someone with Alzheimer's disease.

NLM is currently developing a clinical trials database that provides patients, families and members of the public easy access to information about clinical research studies [30]. The project was initiated as a result of the Food and Drug Administration (FDA) Modernization Act of November 1997 which requires the establishment of a registry of clinical trials for experimental treatments for serious or life-threatening diseases [31]. The system will be a comprehensive resource that includes clinical studies funded by the U.S. Federal government and by private industry. At some future time, international studies may also be included. The database will include summaries of the purpose of each clinical research study, together with the recruiting status, the criteria for patient participation in the trial, the location of the trial, and specific contact information. Other information in the database includes the research study design, the phase of the trial, the disease or condition, and the particular drug or therapy under study.

An important feature of the clinical trials database will be to provide access to other online health resources that help place a clinical trial in the context of a patient's overall medical care. For example, an ongoing clinical trial on age-related macular degeneration would be linked to organizations that might have information on this vision disorder, including the American Academy of Ophthalmology and the Macular Degeneration Foundation, as well as the trial's sponsoring organization, in this case, the National Eye Institute (NEI). NEI has developed information resources for patients with age-related macular degeneration which answer questions such as "What is the macula?"; "Who is at risk for age-related macular degeneration?"; "How is the disease treated?"; and "What research is being done?" (http://www.nei.nih.gov/publications/armd-p.htm). Since one of the MEDLINE*plus* topics is macular degeneration, interested individuals would also be able to find information on prevention and screening for the disease as well as nutritional advice. If desired, at this point a PubMed search for a review of age-related macular degeneration could be run and this would result in several current articles on the topic.

5. Conclusions

Internet technology and its promise have raised many technical as well as social and economic issues. The increasingly complex information environment, in which we live and work, requires us to modify old models and develop new ones for managing information creation and use. Content and interfaces must be designed to adequately serve a broad range of potential audiences. Effective methods for searching and navigating multiple sources of information are needed, so that seamless and intuitive access to the information we have created is provided. Nowhere is this more important than in health care.

The medical informatics community has long been concerned with the effective use of computers for improving health care. World Wide Web technology, though in many ways still in its infancy, and, in spite of its obvious deficiencies, has revolutionized the way people are seeking and using information. Our discipline is well positioned to transfer the research and thinking we have done about information creation, management, and dissemination to this new and ever-growing information environment. We need to participate in the research, and we have the responsibility, not only as informatics researchers, but also as educated citizens, to engage in the dialogue about the many social, economic, and policy implications raised by Internet technology. As Lesk notes, "Digital libraries are going to change the social system by which information is collected and transferred... We need to decide how the typical citizen will get information, how important information transfer is to democracy, and how we will preserve the accessibility of information that we want and the diversity that we would like" [32].

References

[1] Lagoze, C., Fielding, D. Defining collections in distributed digital libraries. D-Lib Magazine, November 1998.

[2] Program Announcement: Research on Digital Libraries, sponsored by the National Science Foundation, the Advanced Research Projects Agency, and the National Aeronautics and Space Administration, 1993.

[3] Program Announcement: Digital Libraries Initiative - Phase 2, sponsored by the National Science Foundation, the Defense Advanced Research Projects Agency, the National Library of Medicine, the Library of Congress, the National Aeronautics & Space Administration, and the National Endowment for the Humanities, 1997.

[4] Lynch, C. Searching the Internet. Scientific American, March 1997, 52-6.

[5] Waters, D.J. The Digital Library Federation: Program Agenda. Digital Libraries, a program of the Council on Library and Information Resources, 1998, 12 pages.

[6] Rothenberg, J. Ensuring the Longevity of Digital Documents. Scientific American, January 1995:42-47.

[7] Smith, A. Why Digitize? Council on Library and Information Resources. http://www.clir.org/pubs/reports/. February 1999.

[8] Rodgers, R.P.C. Searching for Biomedical Information on the World Wide Web. Journal of Medical Practice Management, 1999, in press.

[9] Sparck Jones, K., Willett, P. Readings in Information Retrieval. San Francisco: Morgan Kaufmann Publishers, 1997, 589 pages.

[10] Lawrence, S., Giles, C.L. Searching the World Wide Web. Science, 1998;280:98-100.

[11] Weibel, S., Lagoze, C. An element set to support resource discovery. International Journal on Digital Libraries, 1997;1:176-86.

[12] McCray, A.T., Gallagher, M.E., & Flannick, M.A. Extending the role of metadata in a digital library system. IEEE Forum on Research and Technology Advances in Digital Libraries, 1999:190-9.

[13] Brooks, T.A. Orthography as a fundamental impediment to online information retrieval. Journal of the American Society for Information Science, 1998:731-741.

[14] McCray, A.T., Razi, A.M., Bangalore, A.K., Browne, A.C., & Stavri, P.Z. The UMLS Knowledge Source Server: A versatile Internet-based research tool. Proc AMIA Annu Fall Symp 1996;164-8.

[15] Bodenreider, O., Burgun, A., Botti, G., Fieschi, M., Le Beux, P., & Kohler, F. Evaluation of the Unified Medical Language System as a medical knowledge source. Journal of the American Medical Informatics Association. 1998;5(1):76-87.

[16] Campbell, K.E., Oliver, D.E., & Shortliffe, E.H. The Unified Medical Language System: toward a collaborative approach for solving terminologic problems. Journal of the American Medical Informatics Association. 1998;5(1):12-6.

[17] Cimino, J.J. Auditing the Unified Medical Language System with semantic methods. Journal of the American Medical Informatics Association. 1998;5(1):41-51.

[18] Cooper, G.F., Miller, R.A. An experiment comparing lexical and statistical methods for extracting MeSH terms from clinical free text. Journal of the American Medical Informatics Association. 1998;5(1):62-75.

[19] Humphreys, B.L., Lindberg, D.A., Schoolman, H.M., & Barnett, G.O. The Unified Medical Language System: an informatics research collaboration. Journal of the American Medical Informatics Association. 1998;5(1):1-11.

[20] Joubert, M., Fieschi, M., Robert, J.J., Volot, F., & Fieschi, D. UMLS-based conceptual queries to biomedical information databases: an overview of the project ARIANE. Unified Medical Language System. Journal of the American Medical Informatics Association. 1998;5(1):52-61.

[21] Rosse, C., Mejino, J.L., Modayur, B.R., Jakobovits, R., Hinshaw, K.P., & Brinkley, J.F. Motivation and organizational principles for anatomical knowledge representation: the digital anatomist symbolic knowledge base. Journal of the American Medical Informatics Association. 1998;5(1):17-40.

[22] Humphreys, B.L., McCray, A.T., & Cheh, M.L. Evaluating the coverage of controlled health data terminologies: report on the results of the NLM/AHCPR Large Scale Vocabulary Test. J Am Med Inform Assoc 1997;4:483-97.

[23] Bernstein, P.A. Middleware: A model for distributed system services. Communications of the ACM 1996;39:87-98.

[24] Suarez, H.H., Hao, X., Chang, I.F. Searching for information on the Internet using the UMLS and Medical World Search. Proc AMIA Annu Fall Symp 1997:824-8.

[25] Galvin, J.R., D'Alessandro, M.P., Erkonen, W.E., Smith, W.L., El-Khoury, G.Y., & Weinstein, J.N. The Virtual Hospital: Providing Multimedia Decision Support Tools via the Internet. Spine 1995;20:1735-8.

[26] Buhle, E.L., Goldwein, J.W., & Benjamin, I. OncoLink: A multimedia oncology information resource on the Internet. Proc Annu Sym Comput Applic Med Care. 1994:103-7.

[27] Lowe, H.J., Lomax, E.C., & Polonkey, S.E. The World Wide Web: a review of an emerging Internet-based technology for the distribution of biomedical information. J Am Med Inform Assoc 1996;3:1-14.

[28] Bader, S.A., Braude, R.M. "Patient Informatics": Creating new partnerships in medical decision making. Academic Medicine, 1998;73:408-11.

[29] American Medical Association. JAMA patient page: health and the Internet. JAMA 1998;280(15):1380.

[30] McCray, A.T. A National Resource for Information on Clinical Trials. To appear in: National Forum: The Phi Kappa Phi Journal, 1999.

[31] Food and Drug Administration Modernization Act of 1997, Section 113, Information program on clinical trials for serious or life-threatening diseases. Public Law 105-115, 105th Congress.

[32] Lesk, M. Practical Digital Libraries. The Morgan Kaufmann Series in Multimedia Information and Systems. San Francisco: Morgan Kaufmann Publishers, 1997, 297 pages.

Information Technology Strategies from
the United States and the European Union
E.A. Balas et al. (Eds)
IOS Press 2000

Knowledge and Change in Health Care Organizations

Nancy M. Lorenzi, Ph.D.
Associate Senior Vice President of Health Affairs
University of Cincinnati Medical Center
Cincinnati, Ohio, USA

Robert T. Riley, Ph.D.
Head of Riley Associates
Cincinnati, Ohio, USA

Abstract. All of us realize that these are times of high change in virtually every health care system, regardless of size or location. As part of this change process, many health care systems are taking a serious look at the area that has evolved as knowledge management. While change may be mandatory, progress is definitely optional.

1. Knowledge Management

Knowledge management - a current "hot topic" - involves the capture and processing of individual knowledge into a useful and potentially valuable form of organizational knowledge. Each person in an organization possesses some level of unique organizationally-related knowledge. The challenge for the organization is to use the collective individual knowledge more effectively and efficiently for better organizational results. There are a number of theories underlying the area of knowledge management, drawn from academic areas such as information theory, management, learning, and cognitive sciences. Also, different organizations will use different strategies as they attempt to implement a knowledge management approach tailored to their needs.

Knowledge management attempts to convert individual knowledge into "what we are going to do in the future" or "how can we do something better within the organization." Knowledge management focuses on the social and technical aspects that enable and empower knowledge and the creation of information. While knowledge management is an exciting concept to many, it is a frightening concept to others for a variety of reasons.

Let us use an example drawn from the University of Cincinnati, which has 35,000 students. The University has an academic medical center consisting of four colleges and the University Hospital, which is now part of a five-hospital system called The Health Alliance of Greater Cincinnati. An information problem arose in the academic medical center, namely, the sense of being caught in somewhat of a trap. The overall university, with its large student body, was not moving as fast with technological decisions as the Health Alliance with its hospitals. However, the clinical and research faculty of the academic medical center need to function effectively as part of both enterprises, i.e., the university and the Alliance. The university systems are needed for many research projects, and access to the Alliance's hospital information systems is needed for both clinical care and research.

To help in resolving this dilemma, the academic medical center established an integrated information task force to develop its information goals. Seven major goals were established as well as technological standards for effectively sharing information with both the Health Alliance and the University. The seventh goal focused on knowledge management. The academic medical center people liked this concept, but the university people said, "You can't manage my knowledge." One non-medical faculty member asked, 'Are you going to strip out everything that I have and take it away from me?'

Without taking time to understand the concept of knowledge management, some of the non-medical faculty members were instantly against it. Their reaction speaks to the major point of this article; accepting changing ideas, directions, technologies, etc., is never easy. When we talk about health care, we are talking about knowledge and the management of that knowledge. To deliver better health care, we need better knowledge and better distribution of that knowledge. Today, information technology provides us previously unavailable opportunities to manage effectively the vast amounts of information available for conversion to knowledge.

We are facing a number of challenges today-including rapidly changing environments-regardless of where we live in the world; large-scale systems are supporting vast enterprises, and there are a large number of people closely involved in our information areas today that were not involved in the past. Larger enterprises lead to issues such as complexity and scalability. Some information systems may be excellent systems for one department or area, but they may not be effective across a variety of similar departments.

The expansion of systems has lead to greater issues of privacy and security, especially as we extend our networks. Today major issues of money and power are involved in information systems.

2. The Issue of "People-Ware"

It is said that the only person that welcomes change is a wet baby! As we attempt to implement our many brilliant concepts, we eventually encounter mere mortals, who often say "No!" I recently talked to someone who is designing an impressive new system (and I am sure this person is absolutely brilliant). I said to him, "This is really exciting; what do your end-users think about it?" Although he has been working on his system for two years, he said, "I haven't asked any of them yet. I don't want their opinion. I want to design it the way I think it should be." Reed Gardner made the following statement in a speech at the 1998 Computer-based Patient Record Institute (CPRI) meeting: "In my opinion, the success of a project is perhaps 80 percent dependent on the development of the social and political interaction skills of the developer and 20 percent or less on the implementation of the hardware and the software."

We did not recognize the importance of the people-ware concept in 1984, when we started the Integrated Advanced Information Management Systems (IAIMS) program at the University of Cincinnati. Actually, this was pre-Windows and PC's were fairly new, so Apple Macintoshes were the most user-friendly technology available. Our group designed a system to be used by the internal medicine residents, who liked and strongly supported the system. We were able to design user-needed systems, although the technology was not yet available to implement the ultimate concepts we proposed. While the residents were happy about the system, the hospital administrators saw the systems as very costly if implemented more widely. This led us to the following change management truth: It is easy to change the things that no one cares about. However, it becomes very difficult to change the things that people do care about-or when they start to care about the things that you are changing.

3. Resistance to Change

Resistance to change is very high in most people, whether they are professionals or not. For example, we can also link resistance very closely to information and knowledge.

Jan Carlson, the former head of SAS airlines, said that people without information/knowledge cannot take responsibility but that people with information/knowledge cannot effectively avoid responsibility. Think about this statement. If people have information, they can be held accountable. In talking about knowledge couplers during the 1998 Fall American Medical Informatics Association (AMIA) meeting, Larry Weed said, "If you have information, you'll make better decisions." If you have information then you can take action. Sharing information will help lessen the resistance to change. It will help eliminate some of the brick walls that seem to be strategically placed in organizations throughout the world.

Sometimes people resist the changers, but other times they focus on the frequency of change. In some organizations, there is a feeling of "change de jour." People in these organizations feel that they just want to "do their work" and not constantly engage in changes that do not appear to have a long-term focus. People also resist changes in the environment, (e.g. managed care), but it is difficult to fight those issues. However, they can transfer the hostility they feel toward the particular environmental factor to your particular change, e.g., a new information system.

Organization changes are also a cause for concern. Is there a constant revolving door of leaders? Are there many "false starts" in the organization. For example, in some organizations the chief information officer seems to think that it is acceptable to train people six months before a new information system is implemented. In one organization they selected a new system and trained the entire hospital staff, but the company went out of business before the system could be implemented. They needed to select a new vendor and retrain the staff-again six months before the system was implemented-and we wonder why some organizations are neurotic.

There can also be resistance to the specific information technology (IT) implementation. People may not like this particular implementation or it may be frustrating to them. In looking at resistance to change, we can visualize a bell-shaped curve, meaning that some people are very positive on one side of the curve and very negative on the other side with the majority of people in the middle being reasonably neutral. However, in some organizations the bulk of the curve is toward the positive side, usually reflecting a positive general ambience in the organization as well as some "wins" in the past. That is, in this environment, there have probably been excellent system implementations in the past. Unfortunately in some organizations, the bulk of the curve lies toward the negative side, reflecting a negative general ambience in the organization as well as some "sins" in the past. This means there probably were past information system failures. Before making systems changes in this latter environment, some general organizational development should be started in the organization or else a lot of money will be wasted on new information technology.

It is critical to analyze where resistance is expected to arise and where it does arise as the planning and implementation process moves forward. It is pointless to waste resources in fighting the wrong battles. It is difficult enough to fight the right ones! Good change management strategies and tactics help an organization to keep the initial resistance at reasonable levels and to identify and cope with the pockets of serious resistance that do develop along the way.

4. Some Change Management Realities

First, change efforts must be vision driven. Second, we need leaders that are organizationally savvy. Third, we must strive for ownership and commitment from both the organization in general and the individuals in it.

4.1 Change Efforts Must Be Vision Driven

You can not just say, "I am going to start, and I will see what I discover." Seeing what happens as you uncover it may be a valid research approach, but it is not providing leadership in an organizational setting. A clear vision for information technology is imperative. If you do not know where you are going, then you are not going to know if you get there. Vision establishes a strategic information direction that is supportive of the overall strategic direction of the organization. A good vision incorporates both internal and external inputs. Internal involves what is happening in the current organization and what might happen in the future. The external vision is collected from anywhere in the world and allows your plans to incorporate the best of the best worldwide.

4.2 Change Leaders Must Be Organizationally Savvy

Information technology leaders must pay attention to the organizational issues. Besides knowing about the technology, leaders must understand organizational directions and politics. In the political realm they need to be positively political. You must know who the power players are-formal and informal-and you must work in positive ways to gain credibility with them.

4.3 There Must Be Ownership and Commitment at All Levels

It is important to strive for ownership by the people who will be eventually involved in the new process or the new information system. We all own a part of the change process. We need to provide the right resources. When change is involved, people are involved. Remember the "people-ware" issues? Are we providing what people in the organization need? For example, for our IAIMS program we hired nurses to work with physicians about the clinical aspects of the program. This was a successful strategy. The nurses were where the physicians were located, e.g. in morning report room, going on rounds, etc.

A system is more than the hardware and the software; it's the people and the organizational considerations. In the past, we did not need to consider the people issues as prominently as today. We were usually not implementing such widespread, complex systems. Also, people were different. In the past people were more oriented to not asking questions. Now they do not stop asking questions.

Today's major new systems require cultural changes, and cultural changes do not occur overnight. Some of the literature on change indicates that from the day a change is started in a complex system to the day when people say, "we've always done it like this", is anywhere from five to seven years, depending upon the complexity of the system. People are often reasonably willing to change, but they do definitely resist being changed. Motivated people can make mediocre systems work fairly well. They have been doing it for years. We have had some terrible systems that worked. Most people can give an example of a system that they know is not a good system, but in some organizations people are using them, and they do not want to change from this terrible system. In some ways it may be their "security blanket". On the other hand, in a negative organization, unmotivated people can make a technologically-excellent system fail.

Our basic strategy is a simple one, although the details may get understandably complicated. You must involve and communicate. While we use communication and involvement as tools, we really seek ownership and buy-in. We want the new system to be an "our" system, not a "my" system, a "your" system, or a "their" system. This is your implementation goal-the creation of an OUR system!

5. A Summary Example

A large, well-known US-based health care enterprise installed a new hospital pharmacy information system in one of its hospitals. The hospital decided that two pharmacists (the techie-pharmacists in the group) would select a system for everyone to use. When installed, this new system was an utter failure. The pharmacists refused to use the system, saying, "Shut it down; take it out!" which the hospital did. In 1993, there was a pioneering International Medical Informatics Association (IMIA)-sponsored workshop in Cincinnati that focused on the organizational and people aspects of technological change. A person from the hospital where the pharmacy system failed was at that conference. His enterprise wished to install a pharmacy system in another of its hospitals. Being acutely aware of the previous failure, he decided to use some of the people and organizational concepts from the conference. He gathered all the pharmacists together and sought their inputs and their active participation in the system-selection process. The system selected was the one that had failed so badly before. It was taken off the shelf and implemented well, and it was an unqualified success. What made the difference? It was not the hardware, and it was not the software. Both were essentially unchanged. The difference was the "people-ware"!

Information Technology Strategies from the United States and the European Union
E.A. Balas et al. (Eds)
IOS Press 2000

Incorporating Knowledge into Commercially Available Systems

Jean Roberts, B.Sc., M.B.C.S., M.H.S.M., C.Eng.
Director, First Consulting Group
Macclesfield, United Kingdom

Abstract. The ways in which a potential commercial 'user' treats different knowledge types are explored in this paper. The issues are dealt with by the pragmatism with which a marketing manager might evaluate an opportunity. Academics are typically motivated by drivers that are different from a commercial 'push'. Thus partnership is needed for a productive compromise; addressing questions such as why should academic institutions let commercial organizations have their intellectual capital. The paper considers issues of hand-over, product maintenance and a continued development partnership, especially in a volatile [Inter] net-based age.

1. Attitudes to the Transfer of Knowledge

Anything, which catalyzes an efficient capitalization on knowledge, is very welcome. Academic, sometimes collective, research can contribute to creating leading-edge market-ready solutions if handled in the appropriate manner. There are many things to think about when taking knowledge into marketable products. This paper poses more questions about the process than it does answers, raising issues, giving an outline of the potential problems to be avoided in the transition process and not necessarily solving them. As the Yorkshire proverb says "If tha' does owt for nowt, do it for thi' sen" (which roughly translates into 'Make sure that anything you do gives you a return from it'). This sentiment must be borne in mind when negotiating any transfer of knowledge.

This paper looks at some key issues and lessons that have been learned. Then identifies the opportunities and the inhibitors against moving from the academic to the commercial domain, while highlighting some feasible ideas for making the most of what already exists. The processes under consideration range from research to a commercial base and to a diffusible product from a research idea. Diffusion is a 'Eurospeak' word meaning something that's disseminated or communicated to a wider audience than that first intended.

As this paper will be available in many parts of the world, some definitions of terms, as used in this paper, are necessary in order to avoid confusion. Knowledge is an entity with many aspects covering what is known; an expansion or new 'spin' on what is known; or also what is yet to be discovered (what we do not know that we do not know). It could be that what is known already is subsequently seen in the light of a new context. It is therefore necessary to segment the knowledge under consideration into the generic types described and then consider how it is going to be handled. It is also important to consider the attitudes and the objectives of those who own (or think they own) that knowledge entity as well as the potential acquirer. As an analogy, Belgian chocolates and Hershey bars can both be categorized as candy, but in fact, there are several significant differences in terms of production methods, costs, quality, potential purchases, and in fact the rate at which those sorts of things can be consumed. They therefore have to be handled very differently. The same applies to knowledge and those associated with its management – there are many different agendas and attitudes, which have to be handled sensitively if the transition is to be effected efficiently.

There is a distinction between knowledge and intelligence or wisdom (here referred to as 'applied knowledge') – similar to the distinction between data as opposed to information. Pure knowledge is inert unless it is actually used. One of the drivers for the migration of a potential product from an academic to a commercial situation is potential usage. There must be a bridge of some sort between the academic and commercial groups to encourage them to get together. Like the chocolate analogy, there may be very different groups of people and different processes involved, all of which must be treated sensitively and thoroughly. The process of collaboration could typically be one or a mix of types:

- Of prescription or instruction: "Give it to the commercial bodies, it is not our raison d'etre here in an academic institution to diffuse things out into the market. We're focusing on the science."

- Or a logical plan built in to the development process, such that the deliverables are taken to such a point in an academic context and then moved into a realistic, commercial market domain.

Some academics see the commercial world as an opportunity, but they recognize that they do not have the ability to capitalize on it. Others have learned the lesson in a painful way - "We tried, we didn't succeed, we are specialists in research, now we have to leave our 'baby' to the big, wide world and go and explore other innovative development options." Academics can also be concerned that the 'nasty' commercial world is going to corrupt their ideas. When the stereotypical people, organizational and product types are mixed, the processes of any transfer becomes more complex. The archetypal characteristics are not manifest by any real persons or places, but the traits still need to be addressed.

2. Funding Mechanisms: Past, Present and Future

Traditionally in pure research there was little obligation to produce deliverables. For example, during the earlier European Union (EU) telematics programmes and initiatives words like 'near-to-market' never appeared. In due course, exploitation became a focus of the EU Fourth Framework. The EU Fifth Framework (1999-2002) [www.cordis.lu] is directed to making the most of informatics applications in terms of what already exists by either a further rollout or actual utilization of the new knowledge and technology.

Some see the end of research as a coming of age where controlled hand-over is enacted. Some attempt to market the work to date themselves; a considerable challenge to an academic who cannot easily become an entrepreneur overnight.

Some of the United States (US) public agencies, such as the National Institute of Health (NIH), routinely put their deliverables into the public domain. Some US charitable funded trusts actually produce public deliverables that have an incentive for tax purposes. Universities also have an obligation to the public purse, but nowadays a dilemma sometimes arises with private companies who endow universities, offering patent sharing and revenue streams. A potential commercial recipient of your research efforts may be seen as a way to reduce the development cycle after the research is finished; a means of ensuring that your research gets the wider exposure that it deserves or crudely, by some, a bottomless source of sponsorship.

The transition is actually a risky business, where the phases are in practice not as well delineated as the glib statement that "research... passes into... development... which transitions to... the market." In moving deliverables from one domain to another, there are maintenance risks that have to be confronted. In-house developers have, for example, a tendency to shortcut on the documentation; often written on scraps of paper. Patch-fixed software amendments to avoid repeat system crashes are typical, often requiring idiosyncratic local expertise to keep the systems running.

3. Protecting Your Investment in Knowledge

If the transfer from the academic to the commercial sector goes ahead, one of the questions to be asked is do you need a secure 'Escrow'-type version of the original product, source code, architectures or deliverables? Escrow is a safe haven into which a copy of the material that has been produced is placed in order that any discussion on, "What did it look like when it was given to us? How has it been changed? I think that the methodology has been changed." can be resolved. If that type of discussion is entertained without having a baseline against which to compare progress and developments, it is very dangerous. It is also necessary to consider whether the purchaser who takes your deliverable actually has an option on any future enhancements that you might do, or whether you would wish them to have. The development may also continue to progress in parallel in an academic form. Would the commercial partner actually want to take any further development or would their version have been enhanced and diverged from what was passed over in the first place, into a commercial robust product?

What happens if the research methodology that was used subsequently proves to be wrong or inappropriate? To maintain viability, the commercial version needs to be able to be varied or enhanced. Is there any residual liability or redress if, in fact, the commercial version has moved on from your initial product? Under the European Union frameworks, the deliverables remain in the public domain. However any commercial partners who have been involved in those developments are in non-exclusive or 'pole' position to exploit the developments.

There has also been to date in the EU little general exploitation of the overall European Programmes concentrating rather on the projects within them. If governments invest in particular fields, then it is necessary to sell the worth of the resultant Programme deliverables back to the investing government so they continue to put their cash up for future initiatives. The projects may market their own outcomes, but not the overall aim of the programme. In a similar way, once you have achieved a return from one research development, you need to keep the marketing channels open to the group that took your previous work, as they are more likely, knowing your track record, to be amenable to investing again when the time comes.

Projects can originate from many different sources - within a country, within a consortium that in the EU could have the potential of 20-plus countries and 30 or more partners in a particular project; or may involve for example some of the G8 nations also. The involvement of a consortium, or loose federation of partners in research, may also make the negotiation of the transition into a challenge. The principle to apply there is similar to that of eating an elephant (Cut the product into manageable chunks and address each separately!).

When a commercial company takes over the deliverable of a piece of research, it may be unfit for release to a wider domain. The resultant product for the market may need to be made generic, taking out the (university) specifics, the research version code tables, the hospital ward labels and any idiosyncratic 'fixes'. An academic development may also need extra functionality in order to facilitate the customization and individual re-engineering for other locations. Injecting flexibility into the marketable product will thereby give as large a commercial return on the investment in 'knowledge' as possible. For example, putting data tables in place of hard code or adding scalable parameters to reconfigure for other situations may be required. Commercial companies will also want to add in 'badging' (corporate image and house-style) - changes which make the new research product consistent with the rest of the commercial vendors' existing portfolio.

4. And Afterwards... Do the Organizations Remain Friends?

There will be ongoing issues still to tackle after the initial transfer: Does the commercial organization keep in touch with the academic institution that was the originator? Should the organization be obliged to? Should the organization want to?

To preserve links for the future, it could be that the commercial organization chooses to endow an academic chair or research laboratory for developments of a like nature or make some contractual arrangement about royalties in recognition for the roll-out of the product that started in an academic institution. Commercial organizations must conversely consider what kudos (goodwill or added value) the product will attract from continuing to recognize the originator on the market product. For example, the UK-originated Barber-Quine statistical charts or a European-derived architecture such as Edith and RICHE which are named after their originators. In practice, the commercial organizations may actually acquire the rights to your work in order to 'rationalize' the competition or to avoid another vendor getting their hands on a useful research product. A vendor who has acquired multiple functionality may subsequently make a reasoned, informed decision about which to push or promote.

5. Protecting Your Interests

If it is decided to develop the product from a research base, dependent on the contract that is agreed, the base line needs to be preserved in Escrow. Escrow in the US is typically used as a risk avoidance mechanism. If the commercial company goes bankrupt, at least the source code is accessible. In the UK, Escrow is also used for copyrighting purposes to demonstrate or document the hand-over status of the entity at any point in time in the future.

6. It Is Not All 'Bad News!'

From the above questions and the issues raised, why does anything go from the academic to the commercial sector? There are many case studies demonstrating that synergy can exist, and those symbiotic relationships are possible. It can be a 'win – win' situation. However, there are other additional factors to consider, such as if contracts are not drawn up very well between the parties, if taxation regulations do change too frequently, and if the market potential and the exploitation plan are not described adequately at an early stage. The EU is positively leading by insisting on having exploitation and diffusion plans in their research and development projects, so that the outreach from the initial developments will be maximized. It is also crucial to communicate back to originating organizations and to funding sources concerning the benefits that they get from having the research 'on their patch'. It will ease the ability to get future academic research funding if successful transitions that have added value to the name of the location, or brought financial returns, can be highlighted.

References and Further Reading

European Union. Fourth and Fifth Framework guidance, www.cordis.lu

Getting the Most out of Health Informatics - the opportunities and pitfalls to transferrable applications systems. Proceedings Medinf96, Rumania November 1996

Issues of Transition - Traditional to Web-based, Health Telematics Education (HTE 96, Corfu), September 1996 (CD-ROM)

Roberts, J. 'Sharpening the input and maximising the output', BJHC&IM, (July 1995)

Roberts, J. 'The True Cost of an Informatics Procurement', in Proceedings of HC95 (March 1995)

Practical Solutions: Better Information for Improved Health Care Quality

Information Technology Strategies from
the United States and the European Union
E.A. Balas et al. (Eds)
IOS Press 2000

Opportunities for Improving Quality in the Health Care Industry

Janet M. Corrigan, Ph.D., M.B.A.
Director of Health Care Services
Institute of Medicine of the National Academy of Sciences
Washington, D.C., USA

Abstract. This paper discusses the current state of health care quality and describes some of the factors that are hindering efforts to move toward evidence-based practice. The President's Advisory Commission on Consumer Protection and Quality spent one year looking at the state of health care quality and developed a set of recommendations to tackle the serious quality problem in the health care industry. The Institute of Medicine has started an initiative, Quality of Health Care in America Project, which is addressing many of the quality of care areas identified by the President's Advisory Commission on Consumer Protection and Quality. This paper discusses the work of these two groups and concludes with key issues in the advancement of quality health care.

1. The State of Quality in the Health Care Industry

Much is known about the quality of care from the two recent efforts that concluded in 1998. Both of these efforts reviewed the literature and convened panels of experts, and both concluded that the quality of care falls far short of what it should be. President Clinton established the President's Advisory Commission on Consumer Protection and Quality in March of 1997. The Advisory Commission was co-chaired by Secretary Donna Shalala from the Department of Health and Human Services, which is responsible for Medicare, the largest public sector insurance program, and Secretary Alexis Herman from the Department of Labor, which plays an important role in regulating employer-sponsored health plans. In addition to the two co-chairs, the Advisory Commission included 32 experts drawn primarily from the private sector and representing: consumers and the disability community; large and small business and purchasing coalitions; organized labor; health plans, both traditional indemnity insurance, preferred provider organizations, and group and IPA-model health maintenance organizations; providers, including hospitals, physicians, nurses, and home health representatives; and a representative from a local public health department and a state insurance commissioner. The Advisory Commission was given 12 months to complete its work. It's final report, *Quality First: Better Health*

Care For All Americans, was delivered to the President and members of Congress in March 1999.

The Advisory Commission spent considerable time assessing the current state of health care quality. First, a paper was commissioned from The RAND Institute, which reviewed and synthesized 75 leading peer-reviewed publications from the literature on the state of health care quality. This literature covered acute care, long term care, and many different clinical areas (internal medicine, pediatrics, psychiatry, etc.). Second, the Advisory Commission heard testimony from many leading experts in the field of quality; individuals who have spent decades looking at the quality of health care.

What did they conclude? The Advisory Commission heard a message from the experts that confirmed the findings from the literature. They concluded that the health care industry in the United States has both the best of care and the worst of care.

> "Exhaustive research documents the fact that today, in America, there is no guarantee that any individual will receive high quality care for any particular health problem. The health care industry is plagued with overutilization of services, underutilization of services, and errors in health care practice... These problems with the quality of American health care present a clear and compelling argument for national action [1]."

With the assistance of the researchers at RAND, literature was placed into three categories: 1) overuse, which is providing a health service when its risk of adverse consequences exceeds the potential benefits to the patient; 2) underuse, which is failing to provide an effective service that would have yielded a beneficial outcome to the patient; and 3) misuse, which includes avoidable complications that arise from the provision of appropriate health care.

The findings from overuse were particularly troublesome. A study on the appropriateness of carotid endarterectamies found that 18% were inappropriate and 49% were of uncertain value [2]. Other studies consistently report high rates, 30% to 70%, of inappropriate prescription of antibiotics for viral infections [3,4,5].

An abundance of evidence was found to support the underuse of certain services as well. For example, among Medicare patients in New Jersey, only 21% of heart attack patients receive beta-blockers within 90 days of their heart attack [6]. Heart attack is a clinical area where there is a solid evidence base and considerable effort has been made to disseminate practice guidelines to the industry. The patients in this study who received beta-blockers had a 43% lower rate of mortality than those who did not. Another study looking at depression found that only 20% to 30% of general medicine patients with depression were prescribed antidepressant medications; among those prescribed medications, 30% received a subtherapeutic dose [7]. It is important to emphasize that these are only a few of the studies the Advisory Commission used to reach its conclusions.

In the category of misuse, some of the studies were really quite striking. One study conducted in a teaching hospital identified about 4 errors per 1,000 medication orders; 70% of these errors were classified as those with potential for serious adverse outcomes [8]. Another study of injuries to patients treated in New York hospitals observed that nearly 4% of patients experienced adverse events, and about one-fourth of the adverse events were due to negligence [9]. Individuals on the Advisory Commission who worked in industries other than health care highlighted that other industries have successfully tackled the problem of reducing errors. For example, the goal of the "six sigma" efforts pioneered by Motorola and General Electric is to reduce defects to less than 3.4 per million. The health care industry is just beginning to travel this path to quality and has a long way to go to reach six sigma [10].

While the Advisory Commission was carrying out its deliberations, the Institute of Medicine convened a National Roundtable on Health Care Quality, chaired by Mark Chassen and Robert Galvin. The National Roundtable assembled experts, looked at the literature, and debated the findings. The conclusions they reached were consistent with those of the Advisory Commission.

> "Serious and widespread problems exist throughout American medicine. Very large numbers of Americans are harmed as a direct result. Quality of care is the problem, not managed care. Current efforts to improve quality will not succeed unless we undertake a major systematic effort to overhaul how we deliver health care services, educate and train clinicians, and assess and advance quality [11]."

In summery, there is a growing awareness of the quality problems in the health care industry, on the part of many leaders, both from the medical profession, the nursing profession, the health policy arena, the research community, the business and purchasing community, and the consumers.

2. Narrowing the "Quality Gap"

There are undoubtedly many factors that have contributed to the "quality gap"-- the gap between the quality of the care that is actually delivered, and the best care possible given the current state of medical knowledge and resources.

One factor that has probably contributed to the "quality gap" is the exponential increase in medical knowledge over the last decade. One indicator of growth in the knowledge base is the number of articles published in peer reviewed journals reporting results of randomized controlled trials. The Advisory Commission reviewed data produced by Elizabeth McGlynn at RAND showing that for the period from 1975 to 1980, there were on average about 509 articles annually that reported the results of randomized controlled trials, while for the years from 1993 to 1997, the annual number of articles reporting randomized controlled trials was more than 8,600 annually [1]. We do not know whether quality of care is deteriorating over time, but we do know that the "quality gap" is probably widening as the evidence base grows, and our ability to absorb it is more limited. It is increasingly difficult for an individual provider to deliver high quality care, i.e., care that is evidence-based. Much can be done to assist providers in moving towards evidenced-based care, including: multi-disciplinary team approaches to care delivery; computer-aided access to and syntheses of the latest findings in the literature; structured encounter forms that serve to prompt practitioners to provide certain processes during encounters; and preventive or follow-up service reminder systems for patients and providers.

Other factors that impede our efforts to improve the quality of care stem from the liability environment, medical culture, payment systems, and the delivery system. The liability system in the United States is focused on medical malpractice, as opposed to enterprise liability or organizational liability. Blame for errors is levied at the individual provider-level, while most experts maintain that the majority of medical errors are the result of systems failures. Neither the liability environment nor the culture of medicine encourage providers or health care organizations to identify errors and to learn from them. Payment methods, such as fee-for-service, encourage overuse, while capitated systems that lack proper risk-adjusted may encourage underuse and limited access to needed services. The delivery system is highly fragmented. Education and training programs for providers do not prepare them to work as a member of a team in increasingly complicated organizational arrangements.

3. The Advisory Commission's Plan of Action

After considering the many factors that currently impede our efforts to improve quality, the Advisory Commission concluded that a comprehensive, industry-wide approach to improving quality is needed. The strategy devised by the Advisory Commission to move the health care industry forward has three parts: establishing quality as a national priority; strengthening the ability of the market to improve quality; and building the health care industry's capacity to improve quality.

3.1 Establish Quality as a National Priority

The time has come to establish quality as a national priority. During the last decade, a great deal of attention has been focused on slowing the rate of increase in health care expenditures, with a good deal of success. But very little attention has been focused on the quality of care. It is important to note that poor quality also has cost implications for individuals, the health system and society at-large. Overutilization consumes insurance dollars and out-of-pocket expenditures that could have been better used elsewhere. Patients experiencing adverse events have more hospital admissions, longer hospital stays, and more ambulatory visits. Underuse, misuse, and to some extent overuse are all associated with poorer patient outcomes, which in turn result in a loss of productivity and higher disability and health insurance costs at societal level. More and more experts believe that improving quality IS the best way to contain costs in the future.

The specific strategy for moving forward through a national quality agenda that the Advisory Commission has advocated is one of public-private partnership. The public sector is a huge purchaser of health care. Medicare, Medicaid, Department of Defense, Veterans Administration, and Federal Employees Health Benefits Program wield more than half of the group purchasing power in the marketplace. Employment-based insurance accounts for most of the rest of the group health insurance market. The Advisory Commission identified the need to create "bridges" between private and public purchasers as a first step in moving towards consistent policies in the areas of accountability and public reporting of comparative quality data.

In order to establish quality as a national priority, the Advisory Commission recommended the creation of an Advisory Council on Health Care Quality. The Council would be charged with establishing a system of national goals to help communities, purchasers, hospitals, providers and others target their quality improvement areas on a limited number of high priority areas. As a starting point, the Advisory Commission suggested the Council focus on developing measurable goals and objectives in areas, such as reducing medical errors, overuse and underuse. The Council would also be charged with tracking progress in these selected areas and producing an annual report to inform the public of whether improvements in quality are evident.

3.2 Strengthen the Market

Strengthening market forces, the second part of the three pronged strategy the Advisory Commission has recommended, relates to the idea of beginning to provide more comparative quality information to the marketplace. During the last decade, a number of Fortune 500 companies that purchase health benefits for large numbers of employees have been instrumental in promoting what is now known as "value-based purchasing." The concept of purchasing health insurance based not only on cost considerations, seems quite straightforward, but in reality, is very hard to implement.

Some large private purchasers have worked closely with the National Committee for Quality Assurance to develop the Healthplan Employer Data and Information Set (HEDIS) intended to provide comparative quality data on health plans [12]. But a recent survey conducted by the Commonwealth Foundation indicates that group purchasers, large and small are paying only limited attention to quality of care data.

The HEDIS reporting system, represents a very important step forward in the evolution of mechanisms to report comparative quality data to the marketplace. Yet, there are some important limitations. First, the quality measures that are included in HEDIS are ones that for the most part can be produced from existing administrative data, and these measures do not necessarily address clinical issues of greatest relevance to either group purchasers or consumers. Second, there is also concern about the reliability of the data, which are plan-reported and unaudited. Third, health plans are not required to produce HEDIS data as a condition of doing business, consequently, they are not universally available. Fourth, as health plans have struggled to respond to consumer demands for greater choice of providers, in many markets, the health plans in the community have large, overlapping provider networks. Not surprisingly, in many communities, competing health plans perform similarly on many of the HEDIS measures. There is growing consensus that to provide meaningful information, comparative quality measurement efforts must move down from the health plan level to the level of hospitals, physician groups and disease-management programs.

To address these concerns, the Advisory Commission recommended the creation of a not-for-profit organization called the Forum for Health Care Quality Measurement and Reporting (the "Forum"). Currently, there are many different and mostly uncoordinated efforts to measure and report on quality. As noted above, the most well known is the National Committee for Quality Assurance's HEDIS system. The Joint Commission on Accreditation of Healthcare Organizations establishes quality reporting requirements for hospitals. The Foundation for Accountability has developed a consumer-oriented framework for providing comparative quality information to consumers. The Agency for Health Care Policy and Research has established more than 75 standardized measures of consumer satisfaction through its Consumer Assessment of Health Plans Survey (CAHPS) [13]. There are also many local efforts underway to report on technical quality and patient satisfaction and outcomes.

What we do not have is a national framework for quality reporting that requires all health care organizations and providers to produce minimum comparative quality data, and identifies core sets of reporting requirements for communities, health plans, hospitals, physician office practices, nursing homes, home health agencies, and others. A national framework for quality reporting is needed to enable purchasers and consumers to select the highest quality plans, organizations, and providers, and to assist health care organizations in improving quality through the identification of best practices. Adoption of a common conceptual framework and definitions for quality measurement would also allow us to better understand geographic variations in quality by "rolling down" comparative quality reports to the plan-level, and eventually the provider-level. This can only be done if there are national standards for nomenclature, measurement and reporting.

With the release of the Advisory Commission's Final Report in March 1998, a planning process was put in place with support from private foundations to develop a governance structure and an operational and financial plan to support this new entity. The Forum for Quality Measurement and Reporting is expected to be operational in late-1999.

As we proceed, we have to guard against some very loud concerns that are being put forward. "Can the quality of care be measured? Can we obtain good data on clinical conditions? Do we have the right risk-adjustment mechanisms? The data are not reliable. These are important concerns that are going to take considerable resources to address. But they should not become excuses for not moving forward with comparative quality reporting. The Institute of Medicine's National Roundtable on Health Care Quality examined some of these issues and concluded the following:

"The quality of health care can be precisely defined. In many instances, quality measures have the same degree of accuracy as the majority of measures used in clinical medicine, to make vital decisions about patient care. These quality measures have been used in a wide array of scientifically valid studies to assess the nature and the magnitude of specific quality problems [10]."

3.3 Build the Capacity to Improve Quality

Our efforts to improve the quality of care will be far more successful if investments are made in building an infrastructure to support quality improvement. The Advisory Commission identified several critical aspects of such an infrastructure, including: research to support evidence-based practice; health information systems to support clinical decision-making and quality improvement; and more sophisticated organizational structures and a competent workforce.

The United States has a long history of providing support for biomedical research. The National Institutes of Health have provided a great deal of support for much of the basic and clinical research that led to extremely beneficial breakthroughs in knowledge, technology and therapies in recent decades. Somewhat less attention has been paid to health services research. Health services research is the area of research that focuses on bringing clinical knowledge and technology into practice. Examples of the areas encompassed in health services research include: the synthesis and dissemination of clinical knowledge and practice guidelines; the study of organizational behavior and its impact on clinical practice; the study of alternative insurance and payment mechanisms and their effects on access and quality of care; and the development of technical quality measures and satisfaction survey instruments to measure and improve quality. Appropriate investments must be made in the full spectrum of research—basic, clinical, preventive and health services research—if we are to make significant progress in improving quality.

Greater investments will also need to be made in clinical information systems. Advances in information technology, most notably the World Wide Web and the Internet, open up many new possibilities for introducing information technology into doctors' practices. Clinical decision support systems, reminder systems, automated patient records, and many other IT applications have great potential to assist patients and providers in moving towards evidence-based health care.

Efforts will also need to be made to improve the ability of health care organizations and providers to confront quality challenges. The health care delivery system is changing at an extraordinary pace, but it is unclear whether we are making progress towards more organized and effective forms of health care delivery. The Advisory Commission noted the need for health care organizations to develop cultures that support strong leadership, innovation and risk taking. Education and training is needed to improve workforce competence in quality measurement and improvement, patient safety, informatics, and quantitative analysis. Efforts must also be made to address the serious morale problems of the health care workforce.

4. Next Generation Efforts

The Institute of Medicine (IOM) is a part of the National Academy of Sciences, a private, not-for-profit organization that provides policy advice to public and private sponsors. The purpose of the IOM is to bring together the best leaders in the scientific, academic, and other communities to forge a consensus on difficult policy issues in an environment that encourages careful examination of the evidence-base.

In mid 1999, the IOM started The Quality of Health Care in America Project (QHCA), a three-year effort with the goal of providing leadership, strategic direction and analytic tools that will contribute to a threshold improvement in quality in the health care industry during the next decade. The QHCA Committee is chaired by William Richardson, President and CEO of the W.K. Kellogg Foundation and includes experts in medicine, nursing, quality measurement and improvement, and informatics, and representatives of the health plans, hospitals, purchasers and consumers.

The QHCA Project will be releasing a series of reports over the coming 18 months. The first will be a comprehensive analysis of issues related to patient safety and medical errors. This will be followed by a series of short reports on critical issues that must be addressed to improve quality including: the role of information technology and quality; the effects of various payment and compensation systems on incentives to improve quality; the relationship between increased volume of procedures performed by hospitals or physicians and improved outcomes; and the changing roles of consumers and purchasers. Lastly, the project will produce a report on characteristics of the 21st century health care delivery system.

5. Conclusions

Our attitudes and knowledge of the quality of care issue have come a long ways in the last five or ten years and certainly in the last twenty years. When I first started working in the quality of care area about twenty years ago, it was hard to convince anybody that there was a quality of care problem that was not an isolated concern. That is not the case anymore. Leadership within the health care industry and health professions acknowledge that there are real concerns to be addressed.

There is recognition on the part of many that quality of care must become a national priority. Absent major changes in the health care industry, there will probably be an ever widening "quality gap" as the evidence base expands with the introduction of new knowledge and technology. It is imperative that we think creatively and begin experimenting with new organizational and financing arrangements and care delivery models, and there is little doubt that all of the successful models of the future will be ones that possess far more sophisticated IT capabilities than currently present in the health care industry.

References

[1] Advisory Commission on Consumer protection and Quality. Quality First: Better Health Care For All Americans." Final Report to the President of the United States. March 1998. Available at www.hcqualitycommission.gov or through the Agency for Health Care Policy and Research clearinghouse (1-800-358-9295).

[2] Wong, J.H., Findlay, M.J., & Suarez-Almazor, J.E. Regional performance of carotid endarterectomy: appropriateness, outcomes, and risk factors for complications, Stroke 28:891-898, 1997.

[3] Mainous, A., Hueston, W., & Clark, J. Antibiotics and upper respiratory infection: do some folks think there is a cure for the common cold? Journal of Family Practice 42(4): 357-361, April 1996.

[4] McCaig, L., Hughes, J. Trends in antimicrobial drug prescribing among office-based physicians in the United States. JAMA: The Journal of the American Medical Association 273(3):214-219, January 18, 1995.

[5] Dowell, S., Schwartz, B. Resistant pneumococci: protecting patients through judicious use of antibiotics. American Family Physician 55(5):1647--1654, April 1997.

[6] Soumerai, S.B., McLaughlin, T.J., Spiegelman, D., Hertzmark, E., Thibault, G., & Goldman, L. Adverse outcomes of underuse of beta-blockers in elderly survivors of acute myocardial infarction. JAMA: The Journal of the American Medical Association 1997;277(2):115-121.

[7] Wells, K.B., Katon, W., Rogers, B., & Camp, P. Use of minor tranquilizers and antidepressant medications by depressed outpatients: results from the medical outcomes study. American Journal of Psychiatry 1994;151(5):694-700.

[8] Lesar, T.S., Briceland, L., & Stein, D.S. Factors related to errors in medication prescribing. JAMA: The Journal of the American Medical Association 1997;277(4):312-317.

[9] Brennan, T.A., Leape, L.L., Laird, N.M., Hebert, L., Localio, A.R., Lawthers, A.G., Newhouse, J.P., Weiler, P.C., & Hiatt, H.H. Incidence of adverse events and negligence in hospitalized patients. Results of the Harvard Medical Practice Study I. New England Journal of Medicine 1991;324(6):370-376.

[10] Chassin, M.R. Is health care ready for six sigma quality? The Millbank Memorial Quarterly Volume 76, Number 4, 1998, pg565-592.

[11] Chassin, M.R., Galvin, R.W., & the National Roundtable on Health Care Quality. The urgent need to improve health care quality: Institute of Medicine National Roundtable on Health Care Quality. JAMA: The Journal of the American Medical Association 1998;280(11):1000-1005.

[12] National Committee for Quality Assurance. Health Plan Employer Data and Information Set. Version 3.0. Washington DC, 1997.

[13] Agency for Health Care Policy and Research. CAHPS 2.0. Surveys. Rockville MD, October 1998.

Information Technology Strategies from
the United States and the European Union
E.A. Balas et al. (Eds)
IOS Press 2000

Information Services that Make Patients Co-Producers of Quality Health Care

Kenneth D. Bopp, Ph.D.
Clinical Professor and Director of Group Projects
Department of Health Management and Informatics, University of Missouri
Columbia, Missouri, USA

Abstract. A new era of consumerism is emerging. Increasingly educated consumers are demanding convenience, choice, and self-efficacy or self-mastery. These educated consumers are causing businesses in a variety of service industries, including health care, to change their business design in response to changing consumer preferences. Increased consumer pressures to change health care business designs are evidenced by a flood of state and federal legislation and managed care organizations broadening their networks and product offerings to respond to consumer complaints about lack of choice. These pressures are also evidenced by educated patients, armed with information they have gathered via the Internet and other sources going to their physician and saying, "Together let's figure out how I can do this myself."

In addressing the entire scope of illness cost drivers that are causing health care expenditures to spiral upward in this country, providers need not overlook the role that the effective relay of information plays in moving the patient from their traditional roles as resource and customer to more effective roles as co-producer and partner in the transformation process. Health care organizations and professionals must experience a paradigm shift in both their approach to providing health care and in their understanding of the new role of the patient as co-producer.

1. Introduction

There is a financial crisis facing the health care industry as health care expenditures continue to spiral upward. However, it is not simply a problem to be solved by organizational consolidation and operational streamlining. To effectively deal with the financial crisis, health care, organizations and professionals must target all the drivers of illness and costs. In health care, it is blatantly obvious that all of the cost-causing behavior is not in the system itself. Personal lifestyle behaviors such as dietary habits, sedentary behavior, drug and alcohol use, and smoking drive up a substantial percent of illness and health care costs in the U.S. Also, environmental factors like pollution and violence in the home and the community add appreciably to health care costs. However, these factors have traditionally been viewed as factors outside the influence of the health care industry. To effectively deal with the financial crisis, the industry must find a way to reduce the lifestyle and environmental triggers that are increasingly driving up the incidence and prevalence of illnesses and costs.

In health care, 20 percent of patients, most of whom have chronic or congenital illnesses, account for 80 percent of the costs. Our acute-oriented health system often ignores chronic illness until it reaches an acute stage. Then legions of resources are employed to pull the patient through the life-threatening episode. This failure of health care to prevent acute stages of chronic illness must be corrected by enabling patients and families with information and support to self-manage their chronic conditions if the costs of the "revolving door" of acute hospital re-admissions are to be contained.

Finally, studies of patient compliance indicate that as many as 50 percent of patients do not take their prescription as prescribed [1]. Studies of why patients do not comply in taking their prescriptions indicate as many as 60 percent of non-compliant patients did not understand how they were to take their prescription [2]. If the unnecessary illness and cost of non-compliance are to be avoided, health care organizations and professionals must do a better job preparing and motivating patients/families to carry out their treatment regimens.

To effectively address these cost drivers, the health care system will have to modify consumer attitudes and behaviors. That is, health care organizations and professionals must elicit increased cooperation and improved performance from patient co-producers. At this point in time there appears to be a window of opportunity for health care providers to partner with patients to address these cost drivers.

A new era of consumerism is emerging. Increasingly educated consumers are demanding convenience, choice, and self-efficacy or self-mastery. These educated consumers are causing businesses in a variety of service industries, including health care, to change their business design in response to changing consumer preferences [3,4]. Increased consumer pressures to change health care business designs are evidenced by a flood of state and federal legislation and managed care organizations broadening their networks and product offerings to respond to consumer complaints about lack of choice. These pressures are also evidenced by educated patients, armed with information they have gathered via the Internet and other sources going to their physician and saying, "Together let's figure out how I can do this myself."

2. Patient Participation in Health Care Production and Delivery Process

Health care results from a chain of interactions between the patients, health care personnel, and organizational systems. In the series of interactions that comprise the service assembly, production, and delivery process; patients play a dual role of consumer and co-producer. As co-producers, patients provide essential inputs to the health care process and are actively involved in converting inputs into health care outputs. Patient co-production roles make demands on patients before they enter medical encounters, during their interactions with health care personnel and systems in medical encounters, when they exit from medical encounters, and after they leave medical encounters.

The quality of patients' co-production performances in health care is dependent on their role readiness upon entering the encounter. Patients' role readiness is dependent on their knowing what they are expected do so they can plan and prepare for the medical encounter. For example, if patients are expected to provide a complete and accurate medical, family, and social history; they should be informed of this expectation at the time that their appointments are scheduled. Furthermore, they should be provided a checklist or worksheet to facilitate the organization of this information. If patients are to be adequately prepared for a diagnostic procedure they may have to fast or perform other tasks before arriving for the procedure. If a patient fails to appropriately prepare for the tests or procedures, the scheduled activities may have to be postponed or the results of the test or procedure may be inaccurate.

During health care encounters, patients perform co-production work in transforming information and/or other inputs into health care outputs. Patients expend mental energy, physical energy, and valuable time in this transformation process. During the diagnostic work-up, the patient is often expected to remain alert and provide feedback regarding sensory stimuli that they are experiencing. Other tasks can range from simple ones, such as keeping still during an eye examination, to rather difficult ones, such as participating in a rigorous physical therapy session. The patient may also be required to make choices among alternative levels or types of services. The mental work required in this task should not be underestimated. Making choices is particularly problematic for the patient if he or she lacks sufficient knowledge to make a rational choice.

Even after leaving the encounter, the patient is often assigned additional tasks such as carrying out the treatment regimen, taking medications as prescribed, changing bandages on wounds, monitoring their condition, performing diagnostic-related work, keeping track of vital signs and symptoms, changing their lifestyle such as dietary, smoking, or exercise habits, and managing their condition to prevent medical emergencies. Consequently, the efficiency and efficacy of health care is dependent on the quality of the performance of patients as well as health care providers.

3. Health Care Content: Relieving versus Enabling

Because of the patient's critical co-production role, health care consists of a mixture of "relieving" and "enabling" elements. These two prevailing, and often conflicting, approaches in delivering health care, may take different roads to preserving the patient's health and well-being. The "reliever" approach is when the provider approaches his patient's care with the goal of relieving the immediate complaint, symptom, or illness of the patient. Whereas, when the clinician provides service offerings and tools that go beyond relieving the current problem to enabling the patient to effectively follow through with the prescriptions and treatments of the clinician, as well as, prevent, or even treat, future problems, he is using the "enabler" approach. In other words, he is "enabling" his patient to manage his own health care. Traditionally, health care has emphasized the "reliever" approach. However, if health care is going to effectively address the individual behavior driven costs and take advantage of the wave of consumerism, the "enabling" relationships between clinicians and patients must become more prominent. A key feature of "enabling" is that it increases the knowledge and skill transfer component in the service providers' offerings. The challenge for clinicians is to find the balance in the mix of "relieving" and "enabling" elements in their relationships with patients, to take advantage of patients' co-production capabilities as well as the providers' specialized capacities to deliver services.

4. Relieving: Patients' Primary Role as Information Source

The process of assembling, producing, and delivering health care involves an intensive use of information. In contemporary "reliever-oriented" health care the focus of the information exchange has centered on gathering information from patients; organizing, analyzing, and synthesizing patient information and medical expertise into a diagnosis and a treatment; distributing information among functional departments and/or personnel who comprise the production units in the service production and delivery process; and generating claims for reimbursement. Because patients are the essential information source for the health care production/delivery process, the most prominent patient co-production role has been to supply information. Clinicians depend on patients providing essential information inputs into the process, such as 1) specification of desired outcomes, 2) symptoms, vital signs, illness concerns, and urine and/or blood specimens that constitutes the raw material for diagnosis, and 3) body and mind to be examined and treated. The information brought into the health care production delivery process by the patient is collected via a dialogue between the provider and the patient regarding the patient's health and medical history, family and social history, the taking of the vital signs, conducting physical examinations, taking specimen samples, conducting lab analysis on the specimens, and imaging. Patients are expected to provide accurate information regarding the nature of the problem for which they are seeking a solution or help. Often this means translating a complex set of sensory stimuli into a chief complaint. The patients' ability to understand their experience with illness and articulate it into descriptions of bodily states and/or symptoms will help or hinder the provider in making an accurate diagnosis.

In traditional "reliever-oriented" health care, the exchange of information between clinicians and patients has been asymmetrical. That is, the exchange has been clinician-centered (asking closed-ended questions and giving directions) rather than patient-center (allowing patient expositions, giving information, and counseling) [5]. This imbalance in the exchange of information between clinicians and patients is further evidenced by research findings that indicate that patients tend to be more dissatisfied about the information, or lack of it, that they receive than any other part of health care [6]. This lack of information not only diminishes the value of the health care "product" but also hampers the patients co-production performances.

5. Content of the Health Care Product

The health care product, particularly the product of cognitive medicine, is substantially comprised of information. Hall, Roter, and Katz found that the level of patient satisfaction was significantly linked with the amount of information imparted by health care providers [7]. Since patient satisfaction is increasingly becoming an important indicator of health care quality, health care organizations and clinicians must make sure that the health care product they offer meets the patients' information needs.

6. Co-Production Performance Enabling

Researchers suggest that in services such as health care where the patient is a co-producer as well as a customer, managers and service providers must recognize this role of the patient as "co-producer" and manage them as they would human resources or health care personnel [8,9,10,11,12,13,14]. Bowen suggests that customers (patients) as co-producers have similar needs to employees, if they are to perform well [13]. That is, the customer's performance is influenced by three considerations: 1) Does the patient understand what and how they are expected to perform? 2) Does the patient have the know-how and confidence to perform as expected? 3) Does the patient have the motivation to perform as expected? The same way that employees need to be equipped, patients need each question answered if they are to be effective co-producers in the transformation process.

7. Enabling: Information Transfer That Provides Cognitive Control to Patients

In order to contribute effectively as co-producers during the health care encounter, patients need information that gives them cognitive control as they participate in the health care production/delivery process. That is, they need to be able to predict the sequence of activities that comprise the encounter, understand the implications of the respective activities in terms of each activity's utility in resolving their illness problems, and be able to anticipate the effects or consequences they will experience in the health care process.

To overcome factors that often diminish the quality of patients' co-production performance, clinicians should provide patients information that will give patients cognitive control throughout the health care process. That is, patients need information, prior to their entering the health care encounter and at each phase of the service production/delivery process, which enables them to know how the service production/delivery process works and understand their role. Patients who do not know how the service production process works and do not understand their role in the process, may scuttle the health care organization's production/delivery process efforts to coordinate and integrate activities. Patients may even avoid potential services that they do not understand or for which they feel inadequately prepared.

Patients, while participating in medical encounters, often have concerns about the competence and integrity of the health care personnel [16,17]. Patients with doubts regarding provider integrity and/or competence may withhold key information, which may cause providers to make errors in diagnosing the patient's problem and/or in prescribing a treatment plan. Also, patients that have anxiety about their medical prognosis sometimes fail to understand the connection between prescribed diagnostic and therapeutic activities and improvement in their health. Failure to adequately explain the what, why, and effects of diagnostic tests and therapeutic interventions may result in less than full cooperation of the patient in the implementation of these activities and may negatively influence patient participation in the health care process. Furthermore, patients that are uncertain about providers' integrity and competence may become preoccupied in monitoring provider performance and may not give their full attention to performing their own co-production responsibilities.

Also, researchers have found that post-procedural psychological disturbances may occur if patients lack information about the impending stresses of a diagnostic or therapeutic procedure [17]. Janis indicates that post-procedural psychological disturbances are minimized if patients receive pre-procedural information, which conveys a concrete picture of what they will experience during and after the intervention [18]. Such communications permit the patient to accomplish the "work of worry" which is considered a pre-requisite for adequate post-procedure adjustments.

By providing information that assists patients in developing appropriate expectations and making the service process and outcomes more predictable, providers grant patients cognitive control over the processes that comprise the encounter. When the predicted service production/delivery process and outcome becomes a fulfilled promise, the patient's perception of provider integrity and competence is enhanced, and the "work of worry" is reduced or at least made easier. By increasing cognitive control, providers remove or reduce uncertainty barriers that may cause patients to hold back (withhold information, refuse to participate in certain activities, and/or redirect their attention and efforts to monitoring providers to detect and prevent opportunistic behavior) in their participation as co-producers in the medical encounter and reduce the patient's worries.

After leaving the encounter, patients are often expected to comply with a treatment regimen and perform health maintenance activities, such as practicing good dietary and exercise habits prescribed in previous encounters to manage their health or chronic condition. If patients are expected to perform co-production tasks after leaving the encounter, he or she should be clearly informed about what is expected. Studies suggest that post-encounter co-production expectations are often not well communicated [2,19]. Researchers have found that sixty percent of patients misunderstand what their physicians say about taking their medications and fifty percent of physicians' verbal statements are forgotten by the patient almost immediately [2]. Thus, by increasing patients' cognitive control, providers can increase the effectiveness of patients as co-producers in the service production and delivery process as well as increase patient satisfaction.

8. Enabling: Interaction Styles That Give Patients Behavior and Decision Control

To be effective co-producers, patients, in addition to needing cognitive control, need behavioral control. Behavioral control refers to the ability to influence provider-patient interactions in the respective production units that comprise the encounter. Researchers have suggested that the medical encounter represents a conflict situation where the patients' needs for understanding and information are in competition with providers' needs to efficiently gather information to make a diagnosis, prescribe an intervention plan, and to persuade the patient to comply with the plan [17,20,21].

Researchers indicate that patient-centered provider behaviors (allowing patient expositions, giving information, and counseling) have positive effects on patient outcomes, while provider-centered provider behaviors (giving directions and asking questions) have negative effects [5,22]. Patient-centered exchanges enhance patient's behavioral control and decision control and increases the patient's ability to participate actively in the therapeutic process. Waitzkin suggests that most physicians would acknowledge their tendency to interrupt, cutoff, and otherwise redirect their patients' expositions about their medical history, symptoms, and other illness concerns to shorten the time it takes to make a diagnosis and get on with an intervention [21]. However, in truncating the patient's exposition (giving of information about their history, symptoms, and other social and illness concerns in his own words), providers may preclude the patient from providing important information that will aid in diagnosis and treatment as well as thwart patient rapport and cooperation [22]. In addition to receiving more information from patients, Orth, Stiles, et al suggest that allowing patients to tell their own story in their own words (as opposed to closed-end questioning by providers) results in patients seeking more information as they are more comfortable asking questions after they have "warmed up" by talking about their problems in their own words [22]. Thompson, Nanni, and Schwankovsky suggest that patients' effectiveness as co-producers can be enhanced by providing them pre-interview information and instructions which helps them formulate questions and encourages them to ask questions [23]. Thompson, Nanni, and Schwankovsky indicate the patients that are provided a health topic list and are asked to write down the questions they have for the physician while they are waiting in the reception area are more likely to ask all the questions they wish to ask, have greater perceptions of control, and are more satisfied with the quality of the information they receive [23]. Kaplan, Greenfield and Ware indicate that patients that exercise more behavioral control (interrupted provider communications or actions, asked more questions, had more conversation relative to providers, and expressed negative affect) in the encounter are more diligent in adhering to their treatment regimen, experience better post-encounter health status, and are more satisfied with the medical encounter [24].

Research suggests that patient compliance is a function of patients having the basic information they need to be able to effectively participate with providers in decision making. Making the patient a partner in the decision making team requires providers to provide information that: 1) allows patients to understand their illness experience, 2) allows patients to be aware of viable diagnostic and therapeutic alternatives, and 3) allows patients to comprehend the potential benefits and risks associated with the respective alternatives. Armed with a basic understanding of the nature of the problem and alternative solutions, the patient then is able to negotiate with the provider a mutually acceptable course of action. Having agreed on the priorities that need to be addressed, they can agree and commit to the task that each needs to perform. Hayes-Bantista indicates that patients who participate in clinical decision making have greater confidence in and commitment to decisions [25]. On the other hand, patients who receive too little information to meaningfully participate in clinical decision making, or are otherwise not allowed to participate, sense a loss of decision control. Hayes-Bantista indicates that non-compliance is one way patients regain control [25].

In summary, to be enabled to perform as effective co-producers, patients need to have role clarity and the knowledge and skills necessary to effectively carryout their health care co-production roles. Role clarity is the patients' abilities to understand their role and what is expected and required from them. This understanding alone is of little use if it is not coupled with the transfer of the necessary know-how that patients need to perform the expected co-production tasks. However, information, knowledge, and skills alone are insufficient to motivate excellent patient co-production performances.

9. Motivation and Self-Mastery Lead to Patient Compliance and Satisfaction

In addition to information that empowers them with cognitive, behavior, and decision control, patients need the proper motivation to perform their role as co-producers effectively. Motivation theory indicates that people will be motivated to perform well when patients perceive that the consequences of their performance will be rewarded, the rewards tie to performance are valued by the patient, and patients perceive that effective performance is achievable [26]. That is, providers must explicitly link the patient's co-production activities to favorable patient outcomes (achievement, health, and/or financial outcomes). Clinicians often assume that because they see the relationship between favorable patient outcomes (e.g., prevention or cure of disease, relief of symptoms or pain, or increased functional fitness) and co-production performance (e.g. taking their medications as prescribed, following dietary and/or exercise regimens) that their patients also see these relationships. Moreover, it is essential for the outcome to be valued by the patient for him or her to be motivated to be an effective co-producer. Patients often are not motivated to perform well because the outcome is not as valued as other needs. Patients have multiple needs, therefore, to motivate patients, clinicians must understand the patient hierarchy of needs and connect their co-production performance to their priority extrinsic (e.g., pain/symptom relief or medical treatment) and intrinsic (e.g., achievement and self-esteem) needs.

Providers must make sure that patients understand the relationship between the quality of their co-production performance and the outcome. Motivating patients also means that clinicians avoid prescribing treatment regimens without considering and addressing the economic and social implications of the proposed intervention. Effective enabling of patient co-production must address the economic and social implications of proposed solutions for promoting health. Clinicians can avoid infeasible solutions by encouraging patient and family participation in goal setting and assigning to patients/families strategic co-production responsibilities.

Research suggests that the clear communication of expectations and the transfer of know-how, although essential, are not sufficient to assure high patient co-production performance. Rather, it is the patient's level of growth in perceived self-efficacy or confidence that strongly correlates with high patient co-production performances [27,28]. Patients' level of motivation and co-production behavior is significantly influenced by their beliefs concerning their self-efficacy to co-produce.

Establishing a relationship of trust is foundational for clinicians to positively influence patient's self-efficacy. Providers can build a relationship of trust by showing common courtesy and respect to the patient, and giving patients partnership status, Research indicates that social persuasion is an important tool to motivate and strengthen patients' beliefs that they can successfully perform co-production tasks. Patients who are persuaded verbally that they possess the capabilities to master co-production tasks are likely to be motivated to high co-production performance and sustain it than if they harbor self-doubts [29,30].

To be successful in efficacy building, clinicians must do more than convey positive feedback to patients when they successfully carryout co-production tasks. In addition to raising patients' beliefs in their capabilities, clinicians should structure situations for patients in ways that facilitate success and avoid prematurely placing them in situations where they are likely to fail. To prevent premature patient failure clinicians must make sure that patients understand what is expected of them and make sure that they provide patients all the information they need to perform their co-production responsibilities. When patients cannot perform as expected, they feel embarrassed, frustrated, and their confidence is diminished. People never like to feel stupid in front of others. Protecting patient self-efficacy requires the transfer of know-how to avoid creating situations that make the patient feel stupid in the eyes of others and themselves.

Another way of creating and strengthening efficacy is through the vicarious experience provided by social models. Seeing people similar to themselves succeed at perseverant co-production efforts raises observers' beliefs that they, too, possess the capabilities to master co-production activities [31,32]. The most effective way of creating a strong sense of efficacy is through mastery experiences. Developing self-mastery capabilities requires instilling a resilient sense of efficacy as well as imparting skills. Experiences in exercising control over troublesome situations serve as efficacy builders. This is an important aspect of self-management because if patients are not fully convinced of their personal efficacy, they rapidly abandon the skills they have been taught. When they fail to get quick results, they suffer reverses. A resilient sense of efficacy requires experience in overcoming obstacles though perseverant effort.

10. Summary

In addressing the entire scope of illness cost drivers that are causing health care expenditures to spiral upward in this country, providers must not overlook the role that the effective relay of information plays in moving the patient from their traditional roles as resource and customer to more effective roles as co-producer and partner in the transformation process. Health care organizations and professionals must experience a paradigm shift in both their approach to providing health care and in their understanding of the new role of the patient as co-producer.

Traditionally, health care providers have concentrated mainly on relieving pain and the control and maintenance of disease. An important element that providers have traditionally overlooked is serving the patient as an enabler by providing the information, skills, and know-how necessary to empower patients to effectively perform their co-production responsibilities to maintain their own health.

In light of patients' critical role in health care and its costs, it behooves providers to offer a more balanced mix of "enabler" and "reliever" services in order to achieve better utilization by taking advantage of the patients' co-production capabilities as well as providers' specialized capabilities to provide reliever services. Often, enabler services are essential to gain patient cooperation and the co-production performance necessary to assure the efficiency and effectiveness of reliever services. Enabler services, in addition to contributing the effectiveness of reliever services, when coupled with patient co-production may also serve as a substitute for reliever services. That is, instead of providers rendering "reliever" services to patients to manage their health risks and illness; providers supply "enabling" services that help patients/families manage their own health risks and illnesses. To the extent that the "enabling" relationship between clinicians and patients becomes more prominent enabling services plus patient co-production may become substitutes for reliever services as illustrated in Figure 1 [33].

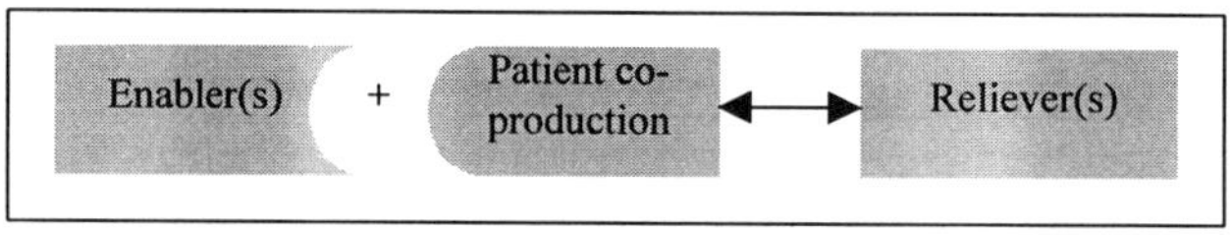

Figure 1: Co-production Performance

In order for patients to become effective co-producers, providers must make sure that patients are provided information that provides them cognitive control throughout the medical encounter and know-how to perform co-production tasks. And providers must make sure that patients understand what they are expected to do following the medical encounter. Behaviors that are related to better compliance, health status, satisfaction, and loyalty are 1) more patient control and less physician control, 2) more affect expressed by physician and patient, 3) patients asking more questions during encounter for more accurate recall of information, and 4) more information provided by the physician in response to effective patient information seeking [24]. Providers that give this know-how and ability to their patients also give them the confidence in themselves to become effective co-producers in their own health care. When patients receive clear communication regarding their role in the transformation process and then are provided sufficient motivation to fulfill that role, patients are far more likely to comply with treatment regimens, to take steps to decrease behaviors that increase illness costs, and to feel satisfied with their medical encounter.

References

[1] Giuffrida, A. and Torgerson, D.J. (1997). Should we pay the patient? Review of financial incentives to enhance patient compliance. British Medical Journal, 315, 703-707.

[2] Boyd, J.R., et al. (1974). Drug-defaulting: Analysis of non-compliance patterns. American Journal of Hospital Pharmacy, 31, 485-91.

[3] Herzlinger, R. (1997). Market driven health care. New York: Addison-Wesley Publishing, Inc., 7-15.

[4] Cochrane, John D. (1997). Year of the consumer. Integrated Health Care Report, 1-12.

[5] Roter, D.L., Hall, J.A., and Katz, N.R. (1987). Relations between physicians' behaviors and analogue patients' satisfaction, recall and impressions. Medical Care, 25(5), 437-451.

[6] Buller, M.K. & Buller, D.B. (1987). Physicians' communication style and patient satisfaction. Journal of Health and Social Behavior, 28, 375-88.

[7] Hall, J.A., Roter, D.L., & Katz, N.R. (1988). Meta-analysis of correlates of provider behavior in medical encounters. Medical Care, 26(7), 657-75.

[8] Lovelock, C.H. and Young, R.F. (1979). Look to consumers to increase productivity. Harvard Business Review, 57(3), 168-78.

[9] Mills, P.K. (1983). The socializations of clients as partial employees of service organizations. Working paper, University of Santa Clara.

[10] Mills, P.K. (1986). Managing service industries: Organizational practices in a post-industrial economy. Cambridge, MA: Ballinger Publishing Co.

[11] Mills, P. K., Chase, R.B., & Margulies, N. (1983). Motivating the client/employee system as a service production strategy. Academy of Management Review, 8(2), 301-10.

[12] Parsons, T. (1970). How are clients integrated in service organizations? In Organizations and Clients: Essays in the sociology of service, W.R. Rosengren and M. Lofton (ed). Columbus, Ohio: Merrill, 1-160.

[13] Bowen, D.E. (1986). Managing customers as human resources in service organizations. Human Resource Management, 25(3), 371-83.

[14] Schnieder, B. and Bowen, D.E. (1995). Winning the Service Game. Boston: Harvard Business School Press, 84-106.

[15] Ben-Sira, Z. (1980). Affective and instrumental components in the physician-patient relationship: An additional dimension of interaction theory. Journal of Health and Social Behavior, 21, 170-80.

[16] Ben-Sira, Z. (1976). The function of the professional's affective behavior on client satisfaction: A revised approach to social interaction theory. Journal of Health and Social Behavior, 17, 3-11.

[17] Waitzkin, H. & Stoeckle, J.D. (1972). A communication of information about illness. Advances in Psychosomatic Medicine, 8, 180-215.

[18] Janis, I.L. (1958). Psychological Stress: Psychoanalytic and behavioral studies of surgical patients. New York: Wiley.

[19] Janis, I.L. (1984). The patient as decision maker. In Handbook of Behavioral Medicine, W.D. Gentry (ed). New York: The Guilford Press, 326-68.

[20] Waitzkin, H. (1985). Information giving in medical care. Journal of Health and Social Behavior, 26(2), 81-101.

[21] Waitzkin, H. (1989). A Critical theory of medical discourse: Ideology, social control, and the processing of social context in medical encounters. Journal of Health and Social Behavior, 30, 220-339.

[22] Orth, J.E., Stiles, W.B., et al. (1987). Patient exposition and provider explanation in routine interviews and hypertensive patients' blood pressure control. Health Psychology, 6(1), 29-42.

[23] Thompson, S. C., Nanni, C., & Schwankovsky, L. (1990). Patient-oriented interventions to improve communication in a medical office visit. Health Psychology, 9(4), 390-404.

[24] Kaplan, S. H., Greenfield, S., & Ware, J.E. Jr. (1989). Assessing the effects of physician-patient interactions on the outcomes of chronic disease. Medical Care, 27(3), 110-27.

[25] Hayes-Bantista, D.E. (1976). Modifying the treatment: Patient compliance, patient control and medical care. Social Science and Medicine, 10, 233-38.

[26] Lawler, E.E. (1987). High involvement management. San Francisco: Jossey-Bass Publishers, 28-32

[27] Lorig, K. R., Mazonson, P. D., & Holman, H. R. (1993). Evidence suggesting That health education for self-management in patients with chronic arthritis has sustained health benefits while reducing health care costs. Arthritis and Rheumatism, 36(4), 439-46.

[28] Lorig, K. R. (1996). Chronic disease self-management: A model for tertiary prevention. American Behavioral Scientist, 39(6), 676-83.

[29] Litt, M.D. (1988). Self-efficacy and perceived control: Cognitive mediators of pain tolerance. Journal of Personality and Social Psychology, 54, 149-60.

[30] Schunk, D.H. (1989). Self-efficacy and achievement behaviors. Educational Psychological Review, 1, 173-208.

[31] Bandura, A. (1995). Exercise of personal and collective efficacy in changing societies. A. Bandura, (Ed.), Self-Efficacy In Changing Societies. Cambridge, MA: Cambridge University Press, 1-45.

[32] Schunk, D.H. (1987). Peer models and children's behavioral change. Review of Educational Research, 57, 149-74.

[33] Michel, S. Towards a fuller understanding of service markets and competition. Presentation, Frontiers in Services Conference, Vanderbilt University, September 25, 1998.

Information Technology Strategies from
the United States and the European Union
E.A. Balas et al. (Eds)
IOS Press 2000

Partnership for Excellence in Asthma Care: Evidence-Based Disease Management

Mary Jane Richman R.N., M.N., P.N.P.
Pulmonary Disease Manager, Egleston Scottish Rite Children's Health Care System
Atlanta, Georgia, USA

Jeffrey S. Poltawsky, M.S., C.H.E.
Community Health Development Director, Egleston Scottish Rite Children's Health Care System
Atlanta, Georgia, USA

Abstract. Partnership for Excellence in Asthma Care, a practical example of evidence-based disease management, was launched by Egleston Scottish Rite Children's Health Care System. The process of development and implementation of evidence-based practice guidelines for the outpatient management of asthma is described. Methods to influence physician practice patterns and the preparation of feedback reports are discussed. The method for measuring outcomes and preliminary outcome data are shared.

1. Introduction

Evidence-based disease management appears to be a key to competitiveness and organizational success in the health care industry. Application of disease management to populations with chronic illness can improve quality and access while decreasing total health care costs. With increasing pressure to report on outcomes and the quality and cost–effectiveness of care, health care providers are starting to implement evidence-based guidelines and monitor their effect on patients' health status, both elements of disease management initiatives. These processes were undertaken by Egleston Scottish Rite Children's Health Care System and applied to pediatric asthma care.

Egleston Scottish Rite Children's Health Care System, located in Atlanta, Georgia, is the largest, most comprehensive health care system dedicated to pediatrics in the world as a result of the recent merger of Egleston Children's Health Care System and Scottish Rite Children's Medical Center. Our system consists of a university based children's teaching hospital, a community based children's hospital and 20 regional centers throughout metro Atlanta where we provide subspecialty care, outreach, urgent care, and primary care.

2. Why Asthma?

With a national ranking of 43 out of 50 on a measure of the overall well being of children, the health status of children in Georgia has much room for improvement [1]. Asthma is perhaps the first chronic disease that comes to mind when considering quality improvement efforts by a children's health care system. As the leading cause of school absenteeism nationwide and the leading reason for admission and emergency department (ED) visit at our facilities, the potential to improve the health status of many children while controlling health care costs is enormous. Asthma is the most common chronic illness of childhood, affecting nearly 7% of children in the United Sates less than 18 years of age [2]. As the leading cause of school absenteeism, it also accounts for a significant expense for employers whose employees must take time off to care for their sick children [3].

In addition to the prevalence of asthma, an asthma disease management project was a worthwhile endeavor for our system because of the significant variation in asthma care and the cost of that care within our facilities. In 1995-96, our data showed that charges for caring for the mild to moderately severe asthmatic child varied by 46%. Our ED physicians noticed a significant variance in the community physicians' management of asthma among children seeking emergency care in our facilities. A number of children seen in our ED were only on oral albuterol which was the gold standard in the 80's, but has been replaced by inhaled anti-inflammatory medicines.

The National Institute of Health defines asthma as a chronic, inflammatory disorder of the airways which causes recurrent episodes of wheezing, breathlessness, chest tightness, and cough resulting in variable airflow obstruction [4]. Long term control of asthma is a challenge for children and their families because of its episodic nature. Children may not experience any symptoms for several months so may neglect their preventative regimen. As a result, an asthma episode may surprise them necessitating an ED visit and possible admission, both preventable events.

The consensus reached by our medical staff, both primary care and specialists, was that the majority of children with asthma, especially those with mild to moderate disease, can and should be treated by their primary care physician. For this reason our asthma disease management efforts emphasize maintaining and improving the quality of asthma care that children receive in the primary care setting. It is our first experience of reaching beyond the walls of our institution to enhance management of a disease. We have experience streamlining care in the ED and inpatient areas through critical pathways, protocols, and pre-printed orders, but the focus has been on care given within the hospital walls. Since the outpatient segment of the continuum was a new venture for us and likely is for other institutions, this example of a practical application focuses on that portion of the continuum. This portion of our disease management effort is called the Partnership for Excellence in Asthma Care, hereafter referred to as the Partnership.

3. A Worthwhile Endeavor

Interest in the Partnership was very high from its inception. A common sentiment among pediatricians was the challenge of providing comprehensive, up-to-date asthma treatment in their offices. Pediatricians voiced concern about their lack of adequately trained office staff to educate patients and their families, their lack of available asthma education materials, and the challenge of staying up to date on ever changing asthma therapy. Thus, pediatricians in our system welcomed the opportunity to improve asthma care in their offices. In addition, pediatricians saw participation in the Partnership as an opportunity to obtain a competitive edge in the marketplace by having outcome data that demonstrate high-quality, cost-effective care. The Partnership offers advantages to other involved parties. Children with asthma benefit because they receive high-quality, cost-effective asthma care in the outpatient setting, which may result in improved quality of life, eg., ability to sleep through the night, participate in sports, fewer missed school days, etc. The Partnership allows our health care system the opportunity to strengthen relationships with affiliated pediatricians, and a successful disease management project will help strengthen its position in the market. The expected reduction in health care expenditures is a societal benefit and directly benefits providers for the capitated share of their population. For the fee for service share, reduction in expenditures makes the providers more attractive to the insurers and managed care organizations.

Given the high interest in the Partnership, finding 12 respected and influential physicians to serve on the planning and implementation team, also known as the physician advisory group, was an easy task. Involvement of respected and influential physicians was essential in getting the Partnership launched. Their involvement set an example for their peers to follow in implementation and change of practice patterns. Four specialists (2 pulmonologists and 2 allergists) and 8 pediatricians (representing 33 pediatricians in 8 practices) composed the physician advisory group which met monthly for 6 months to plan the plan and implement the Partnership. The project was coordinated by a pediatric nurse practitioner with expertise in asthma and the system medical director for medical management provided administrative oversight. A health care consultant also provided support during the planning and implementation phase. The physician advisory group launched the Partnership with the following objectives:

- Improve patient outcomes and increase patient and family satisfaction with asthma care by ensuring that patients receive clinical services that have been successfully tested in controlled clinical studies and recommended by experts to improve health status.
- Reduce costs of care by promoting evidence-based medicine, eg., focusing only on those clinical activities that have been demonstrated to change outcomes and eliminating unsubstantiated or otherwise ineffective activities.
- Support marketing of pediatric health care by documenting better and broader implementation of the latest and scientifically validated recommendations and by documenting superior outcomes resulting from those practices.

4. Development of Evidence-based Practice Guidelines

Physicians in our system had experience with developing guidelines, protocols, and pre-printed orders. Typically these were based on physician preference and past experience. In other words, physicians had experience reaching a consensus on the usual way of care within our system, with little regard to what the literature cited as interventions that have a positive impact on patient outcomes. The result was the stimulation of reduced variances in practice around usual practice. This is in contrast to evidence-based guidelines that stimulate a reduction in practice variances around optimal practice [5]. The idea of evidence-based medicine was a new one for many of our physicians and is defined in the following manner: “Evidence-based medicine involves integrating current best evidence with clinical expertise, pathophysiological knowledge, and patient preferences in making decisions about the care of patients." [5]. Evidence-based practice guidelines are a primary tool for developing an evidence-based disease management program and may magnify the positive impact of the guidelines. Gradually, the physicians in the advisory group accepted the idea that their personal experience and preference may not result in significant improvements in the health status of children with asthma.

This acceptance was reinforced by an extensive review of the literature conducted by the consultant that resulted in numerous randomized controlled trials supporting various interventions for asthma care. The physician advisory group then discussed the trials and those that were not applicable to our setting or were not feasible to carry out in a busy pediatric practice were deleted. For example, family therapy is an intervention with much evidence to support its positive effect on outcomes. However, the physicians determined that it was not an appropriate intervention for their setting but rather an appropriate referral. The process of reviewing controlled trials took over 3 months, longer than expected. The physicians readily agreed with the trials that support the effectiveness of asthma education for example however disagreed on how that education should be conducted in an outpatient setting. As a result, the consultant conducted a more focused literature search on the details of an effective asthma education program.

In addition to eliminating unrealistic evidence-based interventions, the physician discussion of the trials fostered local buy-in to the evolving guidelines, a necessary component for successful implementation. Further local buy-in was obtained by seeking input on the evolving guidelines from other pediatricians in the community. Circulating drafts of the guidelines helps to promote a sense of ownership that may increase the likelihood of later compliance with them. This was an important step since one of the long-term goals of the Partnership is to include more physicians in the Partnership.

Other ingredients of evidence-based medicine are clinical expertise and patient preference [5]. The physician advisory group looked to the Expert Panel Report II: Guidelines for Diagnosis and Management of Asthma and the specialists in the group to validate the evidence [4]. While the physician advisory group felt that they had identified all relevant issues around outpatient asthma management with evidence and clinical expertise to support them, they valued consumer insight and wanted to hear consumers' perspectives on asthma management in the community. Consumer validation or patient preference was obtained by appointing a focus group consisting of eight parents of children with varying severity levels of asthma and one teenage patient with severe asthma. The group repeatedly talked about lack of adequate asthma education in pediatricians' offices, lack of insurance coverage for equipment, and lack of consensus on asthma treatment among doctors in the same practice. One mother's comment exemplifies this sentiment as she stated, "Within the group there are too many conflicting ideas on how to handle asthma. This becomes a problem when, during anything other than a routine visit, you must see a different physician." The focus group provided valuable insight that was used to develop an asthma education program for pediatricians' offices (discussed later in the chapter) and stimulated an investigation into insurance coverage of spacers and peak flow meters for children.

Table 1: Suggested Practice Guidelines for Outpatient Management of the Child with Asthma

A.	**Asthma Education**
1.	Patients with mild intermittent or mild persistent asthma and their parents receive basic education on asthma management.
2.	Patients with moderate or severe persistent asthma receive comprehensive 18 point asthma education.
B.	**Control of Environmental Factors**
1.	All patients get an appropriate environmental screening to identify possible allergens.
2.	All patients receive specific recommendations to avoid or reduce exposure to known allergens that increase the frequency and severity of exacerbations.
3.	Smoking parents of children with asthma get referred to a series of counseling sessions on smoking cessation.
4.	Patients diagnosed with moderate or severe persistent asthma get the influenza vaccination yearly.
C.	**Effective drug treatment**
1.	Patients with moderate and severe persistent asthma get anti-inflammatory maintenance treatment.
2.	All patients with asthma get appropriate quick relief medication to manage episodes.
3.	Patients with exercise induced asthma get appropriate prevention with albuterol or cromolyn sodium.
4.	All patients with asthma get a spacer device (if on MDI) with demonstration of its proper use.
D.	**Regular Professional Care**
1.	Patients with moderate and severe persistent asthma get regular (at least every 3 months) supervision, support, and review of home management plan by a clinician knowledgeable about asthma.
2.	Patients over age 5 with asthma who take daily medications monitor peak expiratory flow rate daily.

After four months of reviewing randomized trials and seeking clinical expertise and consumer validation, the physician advisory group revealed 12 evidence-based guidelines for the outpatient management of asthma. These are listed in Table 1. Severity classification and referral to a specialist are not addressed in the guidelines as the advisory group decided to adopt the recommendations for those issues from the Expert Panel Report II: Guidelines for the Diagnosis and Management of Asthma. After reading Table 1, anyone with knowledge of asthma care will conclude that the guidelines are essentially basic asthma care. However, many pediatricians in our community have room for improvement in the quality of asthma care delivered as will be demonstrated in the results section. This is consistent with studies in the literature which have demonstrated that providers often underutilize guidelines and that patients' health status could be improved, for example, if their providers prescribed more anti-inflammatory medicines [6,7].

5. An Evidence-based Search for Ways to Influence Physician Practice Patterns

Once consensus had been reached on the evidence-based guidelines, the members of the advisory group were eager to put them into practice. Six pediatricians, all members of the advisory group, took the opportunity for their practices, which represent 29 primary care providers, to be among the first groups to participate in the Partnership. The next step was selling their colleagues on the guidelines. For some providers, the idea of practice guidelines may conjure up images of "cookbook medicine" or the loss of independent decision-making regarding patient care. However this perception was largely averted in our Partnership for a number of reasons. First, the guidelines were developed by practicing physicians, not administrators or insurance companies, and were based on randomized controlled trials, the gold standard of scientific evidence. Thus the credibility of the guidelines was high.

A second reason that the guidelines were embraced is that physicians were involved in deciding which methods worked best to influence their peers to adopt the guidelines. The advisory group reviewed a table of 38 interventions that have been demonstrated in randomized controlled trials to effectively influence clinical practice patterns. A discussion of the feasibility and practicality of these interventions in our setting followed, similar to that with the guidelines. Examples of methods that the advisory group used for the Partnership include reading materials targeting specific practice recommendations (with key points highlighted), reminder stickers with the guidelines attached to the front of charts, continuing medical education offerings, brief personal educational visits by a clinical pharmacist or colleague on a particular drug or treatment (known as academic detailing), and feedback reports profiling utilization of guidelines.

Providing physicians with feedback on their practice patterns in which they are compared to their colleagues may motivate a change in behavior [8]. Giving physicians comparative information on their practice patterns appeals to many of the common personality traits of physicians – competitive, factual, and driven by success. Thus, data that show a physician as an outlier may stimulate that physician to change his behavior [8]. In addition, practice pattern feedback may identify areas where the guidelines need to be modified. Baseline practice patterns were assessed, using the guidelines as the standard of care, by the project coordinator who reviewed approximately 10 asthma charts per physician in each of the 6 participating practices. Data were entered directly into a database on a laptop computer to allow for easy preparation of feedback reports. Reports were created for each practice that compared each physician to his or her peers and to the aggregate group (all 29 participating physicians). Reporting was blinded. Per the physicians' request, the format of the reports was color-coded bar graphs that allowed for quick identification. Chart reviews were conducted and data reported in a similar manner after 6 months of guideline implementation. This process will be repeated after 1 year of guideline implementation.

Early involvement of respected and influential physicians is an another reason that the guidelines were embraced. The advisory group consisted of opinion leaders so that their adoption of the guidelines set a strong example for their peers to follow. In addition, there was unanimous agreement among the advisory group that every child with asthma should be treated according to the guidelines. The hospital agreed to share its resources with pediatricians to ensure that the guidelines could be easily implemented in a busy pediatric office. This reinforced the true partnership for improved asthma care between pediatricians and the hospital. This supportive relationship helped entice physicians to participate in the Partnership and embrace the guidelines. With the exception of academic detailing, all of the above interventions for influencing physician practice patterns were used throughout the implementation phase of the Partnership. Ongoing intervention is necessary because physicians tend to return to their usual practice patterns unless they are continuously reminded of the guidelines [8].

6. Measuring Outcomes

The outcome objectives of the Partnership identify what scientifically sound interventions and superior quality care should mean to the health status of children with asthma and their families:

- Reduced annual hospitalization rate
- Shorter average length of stay among children who are admitted
- Reduced annual number of ED visits
- Lower rate of school absenteeism
- Lower rate of parent absence from work due to child's asthma
- Improved quality of life

Our health care system and the participating pediatric practices are not on the same computer network so collection of outcome data electronically was not an option. In addition, patients of these physicians may seek ED care and admissions at facilities other than ours. Therefore, a 10-question, multiple choice questionnaire was developed that was mailed to families in order to collect data. For quality of life outcomes, the questionnaire contains 3 questions about the degree that asthma interferes with sports, usual daily activities, and the child's emotional state and 2 questions about number of school days and parent workdays missed due to asthma. To assess health care utilization, questions are included regarding number of ED visits and unplanned doctor's office visits due to asthma in the past 6 months, and the number of admissions and number of nights spent in the hospital in the last 6 months. Lastly, there are 2 questions about parents' assessment of child's health and satisfaction with asthma care received.

Prior to actually utilizing the guidelines in practice, each participating practice provided the coordinator with 100 - 150 randomly chosen names and addresses of children with asthma. The questionnaire was mailed to these families in order to obtain a baseline health status of the population. A personalized cover letter from the primary care physician accompanied the questionnaire explaining their participation in the project and that our facility would be analyzing the data. The letter contained implied consent as it stated that by returning the questionnaire the parent was indicating willingness to provide the requested information. A self-addressed stamped return envelope was also included with the questionnaire. Results were anonymous; there were no names or identification numbers on the questionnaire. Results from the questionnaire were entered into a database, and reports were generated for each practice demonstrating the baseline health status of a sample of their patients with asthma.

After the guidelines had been utilized in practice for 6 months, the same questionnaire was mailed to another random group of patients who had been seen for asthma during the prior 6 months. The questionnaire will be mailed again when the guidelines have been utilized for 1 year. It is appropriate to mail to a different group of patients at each interval because our aim is to measure a change in the health status of a population of children with asthma. We realize this may introduce an element of selection, since asthma patients may leave or come into a practice because of the Partnership system for management.

7. Using the Guidelines in a Busy Pediatric Office

While the physician advisory group agreed with the practice guidelines and was eager to implement them, it was apparent that the hospital needed to ensure that the guidelines were as user friendly as possible. Numerous national organizations have produced guidelines, and we have learned from previous experience that within our system they are rarely put into practice because they are too cumbersome to interpret and apply. Given the high volume of patients seen daily by the participating providers and their concerns about inadequate asthma education resources in their offices, the hospital shared some of its materials and staff resources to assist pediatricians in utilizing the guidelines.

Asthma education was the area for which pediatricians sought the most assistance. The hospital was willing to share previously developed parent and child asthma education material, such as teaching sheets on each of the medications; a packet of information entitled "Asthma Basics", which covers pathophysiology, triggers, early warning signs, signs of distress, and resources; and an accompanying video. In fact, it was seen as an advantage to have our education material in the community because it ensured that parents and children received a consistent message. The pediatricians also identified a need to have their office staff trained to conduct asthma education sessions. Previously the doctors tried to squeeze in bits of education during an office visit and often had a limited number of staff, if any, who were comfortable reviewing inhaler technique, etc, with the child. The hospital's Asthma Center for Education responded by developing an asthma education program for office staff, known as ACE Asthma. The program includes a flip chart of visual teaching aids, a resource manual for office staff, and a simplified management plan based on the green, yellow, and red zone system. An asthma educator from the hospital spends several hours with each practice training the staff on how to conduct basic asthma education sessions in their office. An expectation of the Partnership was that all participating practices would become proficient in providing basic asthma education for their patients. The 18-point education program mentioned in the guidelines is more comprehensive, and offices were given the option of having designated staff become proficient in comprehensive education. Alternatively, offices may refer children to an outpatient comprehensive education program at our facility that has been in place since 1994.

Physicians also sought assistance with implementing the guideline related to referring parents to smoking cessation programs. None of the pediatricians disagreed with the recommendation, however they requested a list of smoking cessation programs to give to appropriate parents. As a result, the hospital developed a list of smoking cessation programs in the metro area that is now used in the Partnership as well as our ED and inpatient areas.

Access to spacers and peak flow meters was another obstacle to adhering to the guidelines. Physicians predicted poor utilization of the guidelines recommending spacers and peak flow meters because many of their patients' insurance plans will not cover the equipment and some families are unable or unwilling to pay out of pocket for them. Similarly, a large percentage of children treated in the practices are covered by Medicaid, which requires a laborious prior approval process for coverage of such equipment.

The Partnership was able to assist with these issues in several ways. First, the advisory group wrote a letter to the commissioner of Medicaid explaining the necessity of the equipment. This drew attention to the gap in coverage and resulted in subsequent proposed reform. To reduce the financial burden of families who must purchase the equipment, the Partnership was able to assist pediatric offices with acquisition of the equipment from the distributor at substantial savings that could then be passed on to the patient. Our health care system's response to the doctors' requests demonstrates our commitment to improving the quality of asthma care in the community and promoting a true partnership between community providers and the hospital.

8. Preliminary Outcome Data

Implementation of the Partnership was met with several challenges that resulted in delay of outcome data collection. Perhaps most surprising and challenging for the coordinator of the Partnership was frequent turnover of physician office staff. The turnover of nurses and medical assistants required repetition of the ACE Asthma training program and re-orientation to the Partnership. Front office staff turnover resulted in lapse in communication between old and new staff on the status of pulling charts for review and obtaining addresses for mailings with subsequent delayed access by the coordinator to the necessary information. As a result, adhering to any kind of timeline or schedule was challenging despite reminder phone calls and explanations to office staff. Sporadic enthusiasm among participating physicians was another challenge given the delay experienced in data collection and outcome reporting.

At the time of publication, the 6-month outcome data was available for the 6 practices. As mentioned previously, physician practice patterns related to utilization of the guidelines were assessed by manual chart review prior to implementing the guidelines and again 6 months post-implementation. The data are summarized in Table 2. Overall, in the 6 months since implementing the guidelines in practice, physician utilization of the guidelines has noticeably increased. These data are consistent with the physicians' self-perceptions of their degree of change in management of asthma. As part of an evaluation of the Partnership itself, physicians were asked to rate on a scale of 1-5 (with 1 being no change and 5 being total change) the degree of change in their asthma practice patterns. The average score was 3.6 indicating those physicians feel they have changed their practice patterns somewhat as a result of participating in the Partnership.

Table 2: Physician Practice Pattern Data

Baseline: % compliance on appropriate patients prior to implementation

6 Months Post: % compliance on appropriate patients 6-months post-implementation

Guideline Indicator	**Baseline**	**6 Months Post**
Basic Education	30%	70%
Refer. Comp. Education	13%	34%
Environmental Screening	21%	70%
Trigger Avoidance	24%	70%
Smoke Cessation Referral	3%	3%
Annual Flu Shot	19%	13%
Inhaled Anti-inflammatory	45%	63%
Albuterol as Needed	81%	100%
Pre-exercise Medication	9%	6%
Spacer Device	20%	49%
F/U with Education	27%	8%
Peak Flow Meter	18%	40%

However, there are 3 guidelines for which physician compliance could be enhanced. Smoking cessation referrals, pre-exercise medication, and regular follow-up of moderate and severe patients are down from baseline. These 3 guidelines will be stressed in future physician mailings related to the Partnership. Similarly, the administration of the flu shot is decreased post-implementation. However, this is likely due to the timing of the chart review given the specific time frame in which the flu shot should be given.

Outcome data related to the children's health status was obtained by mailing a questionnaire to the parents of children with asthma whose addresses were provided by the pediatricians' offices. For the baseline mailing, the return rate was 50% (114/228) and at 6-months post implementation, the return rate was 50% (158/317). Characteristics of the population sampling at baseline compared to 6-months post-implementation are summarized in Table 3. The most notable change since baseline is the decrease in number of parents reporting no unplanned office visits for asthma. We do not view this as a negative outcome, as we would rather see parents seek unplanned asthma care in the PCP office than the ED. The population of children sampled at 6-months post-implementation does not reveal a marked improvement in health status since their pediatricians began participating in the Partnership. This may be partially explained by the seasonality of asthma and the timing of mailing the questionnaires. Typically children with asthma suffer more attacks in the winter months so one might expect a slightly higher health care resource utilization rate and a slightly lower quality of life for asthma sufferers in the winter months.

Table 3: Health Status Outcomes of Children with Asthma

Baseline: Results of health status questionnaires sent prior to implementing guidelines.

6 Months Post: Results of health status questionnaires sent 6 months after implementing guidelines.

Health Status Indicator	**Baseline**	**6 Months Post**
% reporting 0 school absence due to asthma in past 6 months	49%	38%
% reporting 0 parent work absence due to child's asthma in past 6 months	62%	62%
% reporting no interference with usual activities in past 6 months	30%	23%
% reporting no emotional problems due to asthma in past 6 months	40%	38%
% reporting no interference with sports due to asthma in past 6 months	32%	27%
% reporting no unplanned office visits for asthma in past 6 months	46%	23%
% reporting no ED visits for asthma in past 6 months	82%	81%
% reporting no admissions for asthma in past 6 months	96%	94%
% rating child's health as excellent	33%	34%
% rating physician asthma care as excellent	50%	50%

Due to the unexpected delays in obtaining addresses from those practices experiencing significant staff turnover, some populations may have been sampled at baseline during the summer months for example, and during the winter months for the 6-month post-implementation mailing. For this reason, we believe the one-year post-implementation data will be more meaningful and indicative of the impact of the Partnership on the health status of children with asthma.

9. Summary

Our experience with developing and implementing the outpatient component of an evidence-based disease management initiative has been a positive one. Involvement of respected practicing physicians in the planning phase, recommendation of evidence-based guidelines, and the supportive relationship between the hospital and participating practices have been essential to the successful launching of an asthma disease management program by a children's health care system. As the 1 year post-implementation mark approaches, we are preparing for the final data collection stage. We envision continued utilization of the guidelines by a growing number of pediatricians and improved health status of children with asthma in Georgia as we invite more physicians in our community and state to participate in the Partnership.

References

[1] Kids count data book 1998: State profiles of well-being. (1998). Baltimore, MD: Annie E. Casey Foundation.

[2] CDC. Asthma mortality and hospitalization among children and young adults – United States. 1980-1993. *Morbidity and Mortality Weekly Reports* 1996;45:350-353.

[3] Weiss, K.B., Gergen, P.J., & Hodgson, T.A. An economic evaluation of asthma in the United States. *New England Journal of Medicine*. 1992;326:862-866.

[4] National Asthma Education and Prevention Program: *Expert Panel Report II: Guidelines for the Diagnosis and Management of Asthma.* Bethesda, MD, US Department of Health and Human Services Publication No. 97-4051, 1997.

[5] Ellrodt, G., Cook, D.J., Lee, J., Cho, M., Hunt, D., & Weingarten,S. Evidence based disease management. *JAMA: the Journal of the American Medical Association*. 1997;278:1687-1691.

[6] Kemp, J.P. Approaches to asthma management. Realities and recommendations. *Archives of Internal Medicine*. 1993;153:805-812.

[7] Grunfeld, A., Beveridge, R., Berkowitz, J., & FitzGerald, J.M. Management of acute asthma in Canada: An assessment of emergency physician behavior. *Journal of Emergency Medicine*. 1997;15:547-556.

[8] Lowers, S. Changing physician behavior requires careful understanding of incentives. *Report on Medical Guidelines and Outcomes Research*. 1997;8,19:7-9.

Author Index

Bopp, K.D.	93
Corrigan, J.M.	81
Gardner, R.M.	35
Iakovidis, I.	23
Lindberg, D.A.B.	3
Lorenzi, N.M.	63
McCray, A.T.	51
Poltawsky, J.S.	107
Richman, M.J.	107
Rienhoff, O.	11
Riley, R.T.	63
Roberts, J.	71